HIV AND AGING

HIV AND AGING

Edited by
SHARON DIAN LEE
University of Kansas Medical Center
Kansas City, Kansas, USA

informa
healthcare

New York London

Informa Healthcare USA, Inc.
52 Vanderbilt Avenue
New York, NY 10017

International Standard Book Number-10: 1-4200-6597-1 (Softcover)
International Standard Book Number-13: 978-1-4200-6597-8 (Softcover)

Library of Congress Cataloging-in-Publication Data

HIV and aging / edited by Sharon Dian Lee.
    p. ; cm.
  Includes bibliographical references and index.
  ISBN-13: 978-1-4200-6597-8 (softcover : alk. paper)
  ISBN-10: 1-4200-6597-1 (softcover : alk. paper)
  1. AIDS (Disease)—Age factors. I. Lee, Sharon Dian.
  [DNLM: 1. HIV Infections—complications. 2. HIV Infections—physiopathology.
3. Aging—physiology. WC 503.5 H6755 2008]
  RC606.6.H5835 2008
  616.97'9207—dc22

                                       2008000978

For Corporate Sales and Reprint Permissions call 212-520-2700 or write to: Sales Department, 52 Vanderbilt Avenue, 16th floor, New York, NY 10017.

**Visit the Informa Web site at
www.informa.com**

**and the Informa Healthcare Web site at
www.informahealthcare.com**

Preface

People with HIV are graying. More than two decades into the HIV epidemic, many who have access to antiretroviral medications are entering the senior class. Aging patients have an additional set of medical problems to be addressed. This book is for clinicians who wish to provide optimal comprehensive care to this growing population of HIV-infected people. Our goal is to cover specific body systems that have been shown to be affected by HIV and by aging. Some of the focus areas have been well researched, and there is a significant body of knowledge from which best practices can be gleaned. In other areas, information is formative and will require further research.

Aging changes the course of HIV disease. HIV infection impacts aging. The medications used to control HIV interact with the changing physiology over time. Understanding the interactions of these three factors may help clinicians provide better recommendations and treatment choices for patients who are growing older with HIV.

In the 1980s, when I began to provide care for those with AIDS, the goal of HIV care was to shore up the immune system and avoid the opportunistic infections that invariably shortened the lives of those who were infected with HIV. In the new century, in the developed world, that goal has shifted for those who have access to and respond to medications. Antiretroviral medications can effectively control HIV and diminish the impact of opportunistic infections. Patients are living longer. Clinicians are expanding from a focus on the basics of shutting down the virus and maintaining vigilance for opportunistic infections to looking ahead at the common ailments of aging and how HIV and HIV treatment impacts aging.

Questions about the intersection of the pathophysiology of HIV and of aging and the dual impact on body systems are becoming more pertinent as more people survive longer with chronic HIV and experience long-term consequences of anti-HIV treatments. This book is meant to help clinicians caring for people with HIV disease to better understand the interactions between aging and HIV and to better prepare and treat patients for the cumulative effects of these processes. It is dedicated to those who struggle to provide care and to those who seek care in these changing times.

Sharon Dian Lee, MD

Contents

Contributors

David M. Aboulafia   Virginia Mason Medical Center, University of Washington, Bailey-Boushay House, Seattle, Washington, U.S.A.

Cristian L. Achim   Department of Psychiatry, University of California, San Diego, California, U.S.A.

Richard Aspinall   Department of Immunology, Imperial College London, London, U.K.

Philip T. Diaz   Division of Pulmonary, Allergy, Critical Care and Sleep Medicine, Ohio State University, Columbus, Ohio, U.S.A.

Ian Paul Everall   Department of Psychiatry, University of California, San Diego, California, U.S.A.

Ruth M. Greenblatt   Departments of Clinical Pharmacy, Medicine, Epidemiology and Biostatistics, University of California, San Francisco, California, U.S.A.

Edward R. Hammond   Departments of Psychiatry and Neurology, Johns Hopkins University School of Medicine, Baltimore, Maryland, U.S.A.

Steven Kadiev   Division of Pulmonary, Allergy, Critical Care and Sleep Medicine, Ohio State University, Columbus, Ohio, U.S.A.

Kenneth A. Lichtenstein   Department of Medicine, National Jewish Medical and Research Center, Denver, Colorado, U.S.A.

Wayne A. Mitchell   Department of Immunology, Imperial College London, London, U.K.

Phyllis C. Tien   Department of Medicine, University of California, and Department of Veterans Affairs, San Francisco, California, U.S.A.

Glenn J. Treisman   Departments of Psychiatry, Behavioral Sciences and Internal Medicine, Johns Hopkins University School of Medicine, Baltimore, Maryland, U.S.A.

Christina M. Wyatt   Division of Nephrology, Mount Sinai School of Medicine, New York, New York, U.S.A.

Introduction

Sharon Dian Lee

Southwest Boulevard Family Health Care Services, Greater Kansas City, and Department of Family Medicine, University of Kansas Medical Center, Kansas City, Kansas, U.S.A.

CHAPTERS AND AUTHORS

Aging results in a decrease in reserves of several organ systems, as does HIV. The systems reviewed in this book are the immune, central nervous, cardio-vascular, endocrine, renal, and pulmonary systems. The book also reviews oncology, which has an overarching association with aging and with HIV. The assembled authors have addressed these issues in clinical terms.

Immune System
Immunosenescence or age-related loss of immune function has been recognized for decades. Sir William Osler wrote in 1898 that pneumonia was the "old man's friend," referring to the fact that many elders died of infectious pneumonia, which was a relatively comfortable passage (1). Wayne Mitchell and Richard Aspinall of the Department of Immunology at the London Imperial College of Science provide an overview of the interface between aging and HIV effects on the immune system.

Nervous System
The cross-roads of central nervous system effects of HIV and of aging are a significant concern. Ian Everall and Cristian Achim of the Department of Psychiatry at the University of California, San Diego provide an overview of

research on the impact of HIV on cellular and molecular neurodegeneration and resultant neurocognitive impairment.

Depression
Mental health and emotional well-being is of concern to many who are aging with HIV. Glenn Triesman and Edward Hammond of the Departments of Psychiarty and Neurology at Johns Hopkins University School of Medicine, Baltimore, share information about the interaction of aging and psychiatric problems associated with HIV.

Cardiovascular System
Cardiovascular disease is listed by the Centers for Disease Control as the leading cause of death among Americans and noted in cohort studies to be an increasing cause of death among Americans with HIV (2). Ken Lichteinstein from the Department of Medicine at the National Jewish Medical and Research Center in Denver reviews the impact of HIV and the interaction of medications and of aging on cardiovascular disease in people with HIV.

Endocrine System
The National Institute of Diabetes and Digestive and Kidney Diseases (NIDDK) estimates a diabetes prevalence of one in five seniors over age 60 (3). Metabolic changes including fat redistribution are becoming a matter of concern for people with HIV disease. Reductions in sex hormones, thyroid abnormalities, disorders of bone metabolism, etc., increase in prevalence with age and with HIV. The medications used to treat HIV may contribute to some of the associated changes. Ruth Greenblatt and Phyllis Tien of the Departments of Clinical Pharmacy and Medicine at the University of California, San Francisco, and the Department of Veterans Affairs describe the related pathophysiology of various endocrine abnormalities found among the population of those aging with HIV infection.

Renal System
Renal functional decline is associated with aging (4,5) and has become a growing concern for patients with HIV. Christina Wyatt of the Division of Nephrology at Mount Sinai School of Medicine, New York, provides a perspective on the renal interactions of aging and HIV disease, including the impact of antiretroviral medications.

Pulmonary System
Lung capacity declines with age because of processes that have some similarities with HIV-associated pulmonary injuries. Steven Kadiev and Phillip Diaz of the Division of Pulmonary, Allergy, Critical Care and Sleep Medicine at Ohio State University in Columbus give an overview of the pulmonary changes seen in aging and in HIV disease.

Cancer

Cancer accounts for 30% of all deaths in the United States (6) and is a significant concern among patients. As patients live longer with HIV and evade opportunistic infections, there has been an increase in deaths due to cancers among those with HIV disease. David Aboulafia of the Department of Medicine at the University of Washington in Seattle and codirector of the Bailey-Boushay House provides a review of the impact of HIV and of aging on various cancer risks.

COHORT STUDIES

Prospective cohort studies are valuable for assessing long-term disease effects. There are several studies that provide data to inform our expanding view of the progressive and additive effects of HIV disease and aging. The accumulating data from these large cohort studies in developed countries enable us to more closely study disease acquisition, to estimate survival, and to monitor risks and causes of death over time in people with HIV who live in developed countries and are able to access medicines to control HIV and reduce HIV-related deaths. Brief descriptions of the major cohort studies follow:

MACS

The Multicenter AIDS Cohort Study (MACS) is a federally funded, longitudinal study of men who have sex with men. The MACS cohort includes patients at four clinical sites: Baltimore, Chicago, Los Angeles, and Pittsburgh. Initially 5622 patients were enrolled beginning in 1984, and another 1369 were added up to 2003. About half of the cohort is HIV infected.

(MACS) Multicenter AIDS Cohort Study Executive Committee—J. Phair, R. Detels, R. L. Huppi, L. Jacobson, J. Margolick, C. Rinaldo
Chair: John Phair, MD
Northwestern University, Feinberg School of Medicine, Division of Infectious Diseases, 676 N. St. Clair, 200, Chicago, IL 60611
www.statepi.jhsph.edu/macs

WIHS

A twin cohort to the MACS, the Women's Interagency HIV Study (WIHS) started collecting data in 1993. WIHS initially included 2056 HIV-positive women and 569 uninfected women. An additional 1143 (406 HIV-negative) were enrolled through 2002. This study has seven sites. Two each are in New York and Washington DC and one each is in Chicago, Los Angeles, and San Francisco.

(WIHS) Women's Interagency HIV Study Principle Investigators—K. Anastos, H. Minkoff, M. Young, A. Levine, R. Greenblatt, M. Cohen, S. Gange

Principal Contact: Stephen Gange
615 N. Wolfe St., Johns Hopkins Bloomberg School of Public Health, Department of Epidemiology, Baltimore, Maryland 21205
http://statepiaps.jhsph.edu/wihs

VACS

The Veterans Aging Cohort Study (VACS) is a prospective, observational cohort study of HIV-positive and an age/race/site-matched control group of HIV-negative veterans in care in the United States. The VACS study enrolled 6,237 patients (half HIV-positive and half HIV-negative controls) beginning in 2002 in Atlanta, Baltimore, the Bronx, Houston, Los Angeles, Manhattan/Brooklyn, Pittsburgh, and Washington DC. A companion data collection on over 40,000 patients provides additional VACS observational information.

(VACS) Veterans Aging Cohort Study Steering Committee—A. Justice, J. Conigliaro, K. Bryant, M. Gaziano, M. Holodniy, C. Rinaldo, R. Browner, D. Rimland, D. Leaf, D. Taub, M. Bridges, S. Crystal
Principal Investigator: Amy Justice, MD, PhD
VACS Coordinating Center, VA Connecticut Healthcare System, West Haven, CT 06516
www.vacohort.org

Other Collaborative Cohort Studies

Other cohort studies have been designed to evaluate specific issues or populations.

*   Data Collection on Adverse Events of Anti-HIV Drugs (DAD) Study evaluated more than 23,000 patients in 11 separate cohorts worldwide from 1999 to 2002.

(DAD) Data Collection on Adverse Events of Anti-HIV Drugs Steering Committee— J. D. Lundgren, S. Collins, N. Friis-Moller, T. Mertenskoetter, O. Kirk, E. Loeliger, A. Rainer, P. Reiss, R. Thiebaut, R. Tressler, I. Weller, P. Reiss, F. Dabis, M. Law, G. Calvo, S. De Wit, G. Bartsch, W. M. El-Sadr, O. Kirk, A. N. Phillips, L. Morfeldt, A. D Monforte, C. Sabin, S. Mateu, O. Kirk, C. Pradier, R. Weber
Steering Committee Chair: Jens Lundgren, MD
Copenhagen HIV Programme, University of Copenhagen, Faculty of Health Sciences, The Panum Institute/Building 21.1, Blegdamsvej 3B, 2200 Copenhagen N, Denmark

*   A European cohort including 23 institutions in 15 countries has followed several thousand individuals since 1997 in the Concerted Action on Seroconversion to AIDS and Death in Europe (CASCADE).

(CASCADE) Concerted Action on Seroconversion to AIDS and Death in Europe Steering Committee—J. Darbyshire, V. Beral, R. Coutinho, J. Del Amo, N. Gill (Chair), C. Lee, L. Meyer, G. Rezza
Project Leader: Janet Darbyshire
MRC Clinical Trials Unit, 222 Euston Road, NW1 2DA London, U.K.

- EuroSIDA is an observational study of about 16,000 HIV-infected patients that was begun in 1994 at 70 centers in 33 European countries and Argentina.

EuroSIDA Steering Committee—B Ledergerber, F. Antunes, B. Clotet, D. Duiculescu, J. Gatell, B. Gazzard, A. Horban, A. Karlsson, C. Katlama, A. D'Arminio Montforte, A. Phillips, A. Rakhmanova, P. Reiss, J. Rockstroh
Chair: Bruno Ledergerber, PhD
Copenhagen HIV Programme Hvidovre University Hospital, Dept. 044, Kettegård Alle 30, DK-2650 Hvidovre, Denmark
www.hivforum.org/cohorts/EuroSIDA

- The Antiretroviral Therapy Cohort Collaboration (ARTCC) is a conglomeration of 16 cohorts from Europe and North America and was established to estimate prognosis of HIV-1 infected, treatment-naïve patients initiating highly active antiretroviral therapy (ART). ARTCC provides a meta-analysis of more than 40,000 individuals enrolled since 1996.

Steering Committee—J. Sterne, J. Casabona, G. Chêne, D. Costagliola, F. Dabis, A. D. Monforte, F. de Wolf, M. Egger, G. Fatkenheuer, J. Gill, R. Hogg, A. Justice, M. Kitahata, B. Ledergerber, A. Mocroft, A. Phillips, P. Reiss, M. Saag, C. Sabin, S. Staszewski, I. Weller.
Principal Investigator: Professor Jonathan Sterne, MD
Professor of Medical Statistics and Epidemiology University of Bristol, Department of Social Medicine, Canynge Hall on Whiteladies Road, Bristol, BS8 2PR, U.K.
www.art-cohort-collaboration.org/

- The Hawaiian Aging with HIV Cohort has followed 202 individuals with extensive neuropsychiatric testing to illuminate some of the effects of advanced age and AIDS-related dementia.

Contact: Victor Valcour, MD
Office of Neurology and Aging Research, Sinclair 202, Leahi Hospital, 3675 Kilauea Avenue, Honolulu, HI 96816
e-mail: Vvalcour@hawaii.edu

REFERENCES

1. Osler W. The Principles and Practice of Medicine. New York, NY: D Appleton & Co., 1898:109–112.
2. Data Collection on Adverse Events of Anti-HIV Drugs (DAD) Writing Group (d'Arminio Monforte A, Sabin CA, Phillips AN, Reiss P, Weber R, Kirk O, El-Sadr W, De Wit S, Mateu S, Petoumenos K, Dabis F, Aquitaine, Pradier C, Morfeldt L, Lundgren JD, Friis-Møller N). Cardio and cerebrovascular events in HIV-infected persons. AIDS 2004; 18:1811–1817.
3. National Institute of Diabetes and Digestive and Kidney Diseases. National Diabetes Statistics Fact Sheet: General Information and National Estimates on Diabetes in the United States, 2005. Bethesda, MD: U.S. Department of Health and Human Services, National Institute of Health, 2005. NIH Publication 06–3892.
4. Silva F. The aging kidney: a review—part 1. Int Urol Nephrol 2005; 37:185–205.
5. Silva F. The aging kidney: a review—part 2. Int Urol Nephrol 2005; 37:419–432.
6. Minino AM, Heron MP, et al. Deaths: final data for 2004. National Vital Statistics Reports; vol. 55, no. 19. Hyattsville, MD: National Center for Health Statistics, 2007.

1

The Immune System

Wayne A. Mitchell and Richard Aspinall

Department of Immunology, Imperial College London, London, U.K.

INTRODUCTION

For over 25 years, the global, scientific, and governmental communities have been actively engaged in devising strategies to understand and combat the threat posed to human health by the human immunodeficiency virus (HIV), the virus responsible for the development of acquired immunodeficiency syndrome (AIDS) (1). This period has heralded many positive therapeutic breakthroughs that now provide regimes that have changed the initial perception of an "early death sentence" to one of "life imprisonment" for many infected individuals. Although an overall cure appears to be a long way over the horizon, these treatment strategies have meant that life expectancy has significantly increased in areas where treatment is available. Consequently, more infected individuals will be alive and will experience the combined effects of HIV/AIDS and the "normal" aging process. In this chapter we will examine the effects of HIV/AIDS on the aging populations from the perspective of its impact on the immune system. We will begin by exploring the factors contributing to ageing of the immune system before examining the potential impact of HIV/AIDS and therapeutic strategies to combat the infection has on the ageing population.

CHARACTERISTICS OF THE AGING IMMUNE SYSTEM

The Effect of Aging on the Immune System

Aging is characterized by a decline in the ability of the individual to adapt to environmental stress. This continuous and slow process compromises the normal functioning of various organs, apparatuses, and systems in both qualitative and quantitative terms and also alters morphological aspects. It means that senescence, the process of growing older and showing the effects of increasing age, is not represented by a preestablished moment, but consists of slow and long-lasting preparation of the organism for a morphofunctional involution, which in itself is part of the normal biological cycle (2). Senescence of the immune system, also referred to as "immunosenescence," describes the dysregulation of the immune function related to the aging process, which in turn contributes to the increased susceptibility to infection, cancer, and autoimmune diseases (3). The occurrence of physiological, cellular, and functional changes has the effect of altering the health and well-being of an individual. This may lead one to suggest that as we get older, the ability of the immune system to protect against invading pathogens is severely compromised.

Immunosenescence

In somatic cells, the process of replicative senescence has been suggested to act as a "tumor suppressive mechanism" with the aim of preventing cells from acquiring multiple mutations that are needed for malignant transformation. It entails the irreversible arrest of cell proliferation and altered cell function (4). As a matter of fact, one of the features of cancerous cells is their ability to become "immortalized," which allows these cells to continually proliferate. Hayflick originally demonstrated the existence of a replicative limit for somatic cell known as Hayflick limit. As cells approach their replicative limit, alteration in their functions was observed; these changes are dependent on the number of cell divisions and not time as suggested above (4). Immunosenescence therefore reflects the senescent changes associated with the cellular components of the immune systems. Cell acquire three characteristics associated with senescence, these are: (*i*) growth arrest, with cells unable to enter the S phase of the cell cycle while remaining metabolically active; (*ii*) altered function, where cells resemble terminally differentiated cells; and (*iii*) resistance to apoptotic cell death (4). Summary of cellular features associated with immunosenescence is found in Table 1.

For several years immunologists have actively studied the mechanisms that underpin these changes in an attempt to improve the physical welfare of the rapidly expanding elderly population. One specific area of interest is the functional effect that thymic involution has on the ability of the thymus to orchestrate the T cells arm of the immune system.

Table 1 Cellular Features Associated with Immunosenescence

Common features of immunosenescence
Thymus involution with alterations in T-cell subsets
Decline of naïve T–cell rates
Proliferation and expansion of memory T-cell components
Decrease in IL-2 production, IL-2 receptor expression, and poor T-cell response to IL-2
Decrease in IL-4 production by Th2 cells
Loss of costimulatory signal CD28
Increased telomerase activity in CD28$^-$ T cells
Short telomere length
Diminished B-cell function
Lower levels of TREC containing naïve T cells
Increased anti-apoptotic function and resistance to apoptosis
Increase in immature T cells
Increased likelihood of mutations
Decrease in ratio of T-helper/T-suppressor cells
Lower primary and secondary responses to immunization in B cells
Decrease in immunoglobulin production

Abbreviations: IL, interleukin; Th2, T-helper 2; TREC, T-cell receptor rearrangement excision circle.
Source: Adapted from Ref. 84.

The Thymus and T-cell Component of the Immune System

The thymus is a primary lymphoid organ located in the anterior mediastinum and produces T cells throughout life, although the number of T cells it produces declines with age (5,6). Functionality of the thymus relies on (*i*) an adequate supply of bone marrow derived precursor cells, (*ii*) a number of extrinsic (endocrine) signals, and (*iii*) a thymic stroma that provides developing T cells with a suitable microenvironment (7). Histologically, the thymus is composed of two key regions: (*i*) thymic epithelial space in which thymopoiesis occurs and (*ii*) nonepithelial perivascular space (8). The organ reaches a maximum size of approximately 25 cm^3 within the first 12 months of life (9). From this point, thymopoietic thymic space has been observed to begin to atrophy shrinking in volume by 3% per year until middle age and then by less than 1% per year for the remaining years of life thereby reducing the capacity to develop thymocytes (10,11). At this rate it is estimated that total loss of thymic tissue will occur by 105 years of age. In a young healthy adult (<30 years old), there are approximately 2×10^{11} T cells of which 1% to 2% can be found within the blood and approximately 50% of these cells are contained within the "antigen naïve" population. These T cells have not interacted with their cognate antigen. Their activation requires a number of steps including recognition of the specific antigen presented in the appropriate major histocompatibility complex (MHC) molecule in conjunction with the necessary costimulatory molecules by an antigen presenting cell. Age-related changes to the histological composition of the thymus culminating in a reduction in the number of naïve T cells capable of responding to new antigenic assaults. These cells are required to provide a homeostatic balance between memory and naïve cells located within the T-cell pool. The resultant effect of thymic involution is that the composition of the T-cell pool is skewed toward memory T cells (12–14).

Generation of T Cells

Production of $\alpha\beta+$ T cells in the thymus is a progressive stepwise differential process in which a small population of multipotential stem cells gives rise to progeny populations. Stem cells migrating to the thymus are contained within the $CD4^-CD8^-$ double negative (DN) population, a population which has been further subdivided on the basis of expression of CD44 and CD25. Progress from the most immature stage, $CD44^+CD25^-$ (DN-1), requires the transient acquisition of CD25 so that the cell first becomes $CD44^+CD25^+$ (DN-2) before becoming $CD44^-CD25^+$ (DN-3) and then there is loss of CD25 when the population is $CD44^-CD25^-$ (DN-4) (15–17). Cells within the DN-1 population are multipotential, while those at DN-2 have lost the capacity to form B cells, but can still produce either T cells or dendritic cells (18,19). By the time the cells are within the DN-3 population they are committed to becoming T cells and have undergone extensive rearrangement of the T-cell receptor beta (TCRβ) chain genes (20). Expression of the TCRβ chain at the thymocyte surface requires a TCRα chain equivalent (21) (the pre-TCRα), and these cells then undergo expansion and differentiation so that they become $CD4^+CD8^+$ thymocytes. These immature thymocytes are the largest subpopulation in the thymus and are located in the densely packed cortical region of each thymic lobule. It is in the double positive stage when the TCRα chain undergoes rearrangement (22) after which there is TCRαβ-dependant selection. Many of these double positive cells fail to mature further, but a small percentage develops into mature thymocytes expressing either CD4 or CD8 alone and is located in the medullary region of each thymic lobe. Only a fraction of these cells are exported to the periphery as naïve or virgin T lymphocytes (12).

In a successful immune response, activation of these antigen naïve T cells leads to their clonal expansion, the generation of effector cells, and the subsequent reduction in the amount and source of the antigen. This is followed by a period of cell death since the immune system no longer requires large numbers of T cells bearing that specific receptor. However, some cells with this antigenic specificity remain to become memory T cells and subsequently enter the memory T-cell pool. Repeated exposure of the immune system to the same pathogen will be met by these memory T cells and will lead to a response that is more rapid and of greater magnitude than the response following the initial exposure. This immunological memory provides the rational basis for protection by vaccination.

Effects of Aging on the T-cell Pool

One of the most notable changes in the peripheral T-cell compartment with advancing age is the decline in the number of naïve T-cell CD4$^+$CD45RA$^+$ being exported to the periphery from the thymus (23) and the accumulation of antigen-experience or memory CD4$^+$CD45RO$^+$ T cells (24). Several studies have examined the age-related changes in thymic output by measuring the levels of T-cell receptor rearrangement excision circles (TRECs) and have demonstrated that limited thymic output continues late in life (25–30). These compositional changes may be attributed to thymic involution as well as other extrinsic factors influencing the microenvironment that contribute to the maturation and survival of CD4$^+$ memory cells (31). The CD4$^+$ T cell is a key element of the adaptive immune response and acts as a helper in the extrafollicular pathway of B-cell differentiation and as an inducer of class switching in T-cell-dependent antibody classed and subclassed outside the germinal centers (32). The activation of CD4 requires the costimulator CD28; the proportions of which declines with age resulting in increased CD4$^+$CD28$^-$ populations (33). The acquisition of the CD4$^+$CD28$^-$ phenotype is accompanied by defects in the CD154 (CD40L) expression thereby rendering these cell incapable of providing the "helper" function for B-cell proliferation and antibody production (34). Lack of CD28 on T cells in the elderly is a key predictor of immune incompetence in the elderly.

Furthermore, the proportional distribution of CD4$^+$ and CD8$^+$ cells is skewed in favor of CD8$^+$ cells. Data from the Swedish longitudinal studies, OCTO and NONA, indicates that CD4:CD8 ratio of less than one is a high-risk factor of two-year mortality in the elderly population (35,36). In a study conducted by Rufer et al. (37), the average telomere repeat sequence length was examined and found to undergo age-related changes. Both CD4 and CD8 T-cell subsets had shortening of telomere length, which correlated with the observed shift from naïve to memory T cells. Interestingly, the most pronounced period of telomere loss was in early childhood, possibly reflecting the repeat antigenic challenges to the infant immune system and the conversion from naïve to memory T cells (37).

T-cell Response to Antigenic Challenges

T-cell responses occur in three phases: activation and expansion, whereby naïve cells recognize cognate peptide-MHC complexes and undergo a program of division and expansion into effector cells; contraction (characterized by a loss of ≈90–95% of the effector population by apoptosis); and upon antigen clearance, a resting stage when surviving cells stabilize and gradually acquire memory cell properties (38). The hallmark of memory T-cell responses is the ability to mount a faster and robust response to secondary challenges in comparison to primary responses. This is due to the physiological properties of memory T cells, which accelerate their responses at lower activation thresholds:

- As a result of clonal expansion, which occurs during the primary immune response, there is a higher precursor frequency of antigen-specific T cells in antigen-experienced animals than in naïve animals.
- Elevated levels of mRNA transcripts encoding effector molecules such as interferon gamma (IFN-γ) and perforin endow memory T cells with the capacity to produce larger quantities of these molecules more rapidly than naïve cells.
- Memory CD8$^+$ T cells express a different pattern of adhesion molecules and chemokine receptors, which enable them to extravasate into non-lymphoid tissues and mucosal sites where microbial infections are generally initiated.
- Memory T cells are maintained for long periods in the absence of antigen. This occurs by homeostatic cell proliferation whereby there is no net loss in cell numbers (39).

With these properties, memory T cells are able to mount a stable secondary response and confer long-term protective immunity.

CD4$^+$ Vs. CD8$^+$ Memory T-cell Responses

Antigen-specific memory CD4$^+$ and CD8$^+$ T cells in concert with antibody responses form the basis for protective immunity against infection and disease. CD8$^+$ T-cell immune responses play a major role in combating intracellular pathogens whose peptides have gained entry into the MHC I processing pathway. They recognize viral and tumor peptides that have been processed in the cytosol and are eventually presented by MHC I molecules. Class I and II MHC molecules are required for efficient antigen presentation to cytotoxic CD8$^+$ T cells and helper CD4$^+$ T cells, respectively (40).

There are many subsets of CD4$^+$ T cells, the most prominent being T-helper 1 (Th1), Th2, Th17, and regulatory T cells, specialized in regulating different aspects of immunity. Without participation by these CD4$^+$ T-cell subsets, B cells cannot undergo isotype switching to generate high-affinity antibodies, the microbicidal activity of macrophages is reduced, the efficiency of CD8$^+$ T-cell responses and CD8$^+$ T-cell memory are compromised, and downregulation of effector responses is impaired. It therefore stands to reason that memory CD4$^+$ T cells are likely to fulfill an important facilitator role in the maintenance and control of protective immune responses (reviewed in Ref. 41). Importantly they are essential for maintenance of secondary CD8$^+$ T-cell responses (42).

Differences exist in the generation of CD4$^+$ and CD8$^+$ effector and memory T cells (reviewed in Ref. 43). CD4$^+$ T cells have a slower rate of division in vitro and in vivo compared with CD8$^+$ T cells, and CD8$^+$ T cells have been found to have greater proliferative potential than CD4$^+$ T cells. This might be due to differences in expression patterns of MHC I and II molecules in these cells or more limited expansion may reflect the ability of a single CD4$^+$ T cell to provide help to multiple CTLs and B cells (39).

THE IMPACT OF HIV/AIDS AND THERAPEUTIC STRATEGIES IN THE AGING POPULATION

The Effect of HIV/AIDS on the Immune System

The human immune system is equipped with several defense strategies to protect the organism against the harmful effects of damaged cells or to combat invading pathogens (i.e., viruses). In the simplistic terms, HIV infects the very cellular defense systems that are required to fight off infections. As described previously, activation of CD4 T cells by the recognition of antigen initiates the production of high-affinity antibodies by B cells. In the case of HIV-1 infection, CD4 T-helper cells are infected by HIV through the interaction with the glycoprotein 120 (gp120). Gp120 binding to its receptor CD4 and coreceptor, CXCR4 or CCR5 is required for fusion of viral and cellular membranes. The presence of gp120 facilitates immune escape of the virus through its profound effect on the immune cells. It is a polyclonal activator of B cells, causing them to differentiate into immunoglobulin producing cells while activating the complement cascade. This results in the formation of immune complexes that are unable to kill the virus but instead shield it from the attack of other immune cells (44). The defects observed in the HIV-1 specific CD4$^+$ T cells functionality occurs before quantitative decline. This is due to the loss in ability of these to proliferate and produce IL-2 in response to HIV-1 antigen (45–47). This most likely results in the diminution of CD4$^+$ T-cell help for effective HIV-1-specific CD8$^+$ T-cell immunity. This defect has been narrowed down to deficiency of the central memory CD4$^+$ T-cell subset (48), and further phenotypic characterization of CCR7/CD45RA expression, as originally described in 1999 (49), has revealed that phenotypic heterogeneity of virus-specific CD4 T cells is dictated by viral load and viral persistence (50,51). Additionally, the virus also infects ancillary cells such as macrophage normally required for the destruction and clearance of infectious agents. Consequently, the infected CD4 T cells do not instigate B-cell antibody production and HIV is not eliminated. Despite the best efforts of the immune system to overcome the newly acquired infection by increased production of CD4 T cell, these also become infected. It is suggested that activation induced cell death by apoptosis following infection (52) ultimately leads to the major destruction of CD4 T-cell numbers that renders the immune system virtually ineffective in the protection of the organism from other infectious agents, a state of "immunodeficiency." In a study examining the effects on CD4 cell counts in primates infected with simian immunodeficiency virus (SIV), the authors Mattapallil et al. (53) found that between 30% and 60% of CD4$^+$ memory T cells throughout the body are infected by SIV at the peak of infection, and most of these infected cells disappear within four days. Furthermore, the depletion of memory CD4$^+$ T cells occurs to a similar extent in all tissues. As a consequence, over one-half of all memory CD4$^+$ T cells in SIV-infected macaques are destroyed directly by viral infection during the acute phase—an insult that certainly heralds subsequent immunodeficiency (53). The same effects by HIV in humans result in an individual with an increased susceptibility to opportunistic infections and disease, and a greater likelihood of premature death.

Parallels Between HIV and Aging

A number of functional similarities exist between HIV and age and their impact on the immune system, which has led some authors to suggest that HIV infections can be considered as an example of premature aging, as summarized in Table 2 (54). The decline in the CD4 T-cell numbers associated with primary HIV leaves the individuals with a severe depletion in T-cell numbers. In young individuals, it is possible to compensate by the generation of new T cells within the thymus. As a consequence there is also an accumulation of CD8 cells that do

Table 2   Changes in the Adaptive Immune System in HIV-1 and Human Aging

Immune characteristic	HIV-1 infection, reference	Human aging, reference
Inverted CD4:CD8	85	36
CD4$^+$ T lymphopenia	86	—
Decreased thymic output	28	28
Reduced naïve-cell numbers	86	87
Changes in cytokine profile (IL-2 reduction, IFN-γ no change or increase) ex vivo	88	87
Reduced capacity to proliferate to mitogens in vitro	89	90
Shorter telomere length in the CD8$^+$ T-cell population	91	37
Increased susceptibility to activation-induced cell death in vitro	92	87
Accumulation of late differentiated cells CD8$^+$ and CD4$^+$	93,96	94
HIV protein effects on immune function (e.g., HLA class I downregulation by Nef)	97	—
Increased susceptibility to common infection	85	87
Increased susceptibility to opportunistic infections	85	—

Dash indicates not associated with human aging.
Abbreviations: HLA, human leukocyte antigen; IFN, interferon; IL, interleukin.
Source: Taken from Ref. 54.

not experience the same levels of destruction as their CD4 counterpart. Thus, the dynamics of the CD4:CD8 ratio is shifted toward CD8, with the resultant alteration in CD4:CD8 balance being critical for the subsequent susceptibility to opportunistic infections and diseases and ultimately leading to mortality. In older individuals, the shift in the CD4:CD8 ratio is more rapid because of the slower reconstitution resulting from the decreased thymic output (55). Evidence supporting this hypothesis comes from a study by Rosenberg et al. (56) who showed that the median treatment-free incubation period is 12 years for those infected at age 20, 9.9 years for infection at age 30, and 8.1 years at age 40. Although in the period since the development of highly active antiretroviral therapy (HAART) life expectancy has increased, the underlying association between reduced thymic output (involution), T-cell numbers, and aging cannot be ignored in understanding the effectiveness of HAART treatment in the elderly.

From the prospective of the CD8$^+$ T cell, primary HIV infection is characterized by a rapid expansion of HIV-specific "effector" CD8$^+$, which substantially reduces the viral load without ever totally clearing the virus (54). It has been noted that these HIV-specific CD8$^+$ T cells do not appear able to fully differentiation but remained in an intermediate state, with low levels of perforin and persistent CD27 expression. This inability to eradicate the virus results in continuous state of immune activation as it is recurrently challenged over time (57). In a recent review by Appay et al. (57), the authors propose that the loss of HIV-replication control and progression toward HIV disease may be the consequence of immune resources exhaustion due to persistent immune activation. This may occur at two levels, first due to clonal exhaustion of HIV-specific CD8$^+$ T cells, which are important to control HIV replication, and second at systemic exhaustion of primary resources resulting in the decline of T-cell renewal capacities and general aging of the lymphocyte population.

A rather elegant study by Kalayjian et al. (58) examined the immune perturbations by aging and HIV/AIDS by directly comparing a comprehensive array of candidate immune indices of healthy and HIV infection individuals classified as being young (18–30 years; median age of 30) or old (>45 years; median age of 50). To avoid confounding effects of comorbidities or medications, entry criteria were consistent with the SENIEUR protocol (59). In both the HIV-infected and healthy controls, older age was associated with fewer naïve CD8$^+$ cells and diminished expression of CD28. HIV infection but not aging was associated with differences in chemokine receptor densities, DTH responses, spontaneous apoptosis of lymphocytes, and decreased lymphoproliferative responses to mitogens and antigen. Age-related differences in lymphoproliferative responses were only observed in the HIV-infected groups. The authors show that, with the exception of HLA-DR/CD38 expression on CD4 and CD8 cell, older age appears to accentuate many HIV associated changes in T-cell and B-cell phenotypes in HIV infection (58).

As mentioned previously, diminished CD28 expression is associated with high mortality risk factor in the elderly and has therefore been implicated as an important molecule in the immunopathogenesis of AIDS. The observation that HIV-1 progression correlated with increased frequency of CD4 and CD8 cells [as high as 65% (60)] lacking CD28 suggest suboptimal in vivo responses to HIV. In both situations, the majority of CD28⁻ T cells are within the CD8 subset. In studies on T cells isolated from HIV-infected persons, telomere analysis and proliferative assays suggested that surface expression of CD57 on CD28⁻ T cells defined the ultimate end-stage cell in the senescence pathway (61). Moreover, expression of inhibitory receptor programmed death-1 (PD-1) correlates with an impairment of HIV-specific CD8 T-cell function and may act as predictors of disease progression (62). Although this may be normalized with HAART treatment as demonstrated by Rosignoli et al. (63).

Therapeutic Strategies to Overcome HIV

Prior to the development of HAART, the prognosis for those infected with HIV was very poor especially in elderly as demonstrated by Figure 1 from the Cardiac Arrest in Seattle: Concerted Action on Seroconversion to AIDS and Death in Europe (CASCADE) study in which comparison were made in mortality rates in the pre-HAART and HAART era (64). In regions where HAART is available it has proven to be very effective in helping to control the impact of HIV infection on the immune system and resulted in a substantial increase in life expectancy. Monitoring of CD4 cell counts is an effective means of assessing disease progression in HIV-infected individuals. CD4 cell counts surveillance figures from the U.K. Health Protection Agency (65) between the years 1991 to 2004 clearly

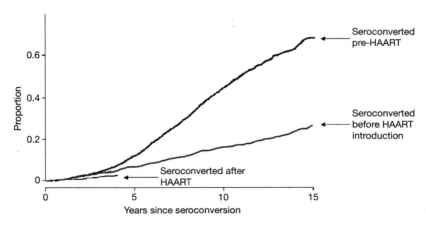

Figure 1 Overall mortality in the pre-HAART and HAART era in the CASCADE collaboration. Black line represents the mortality in the pre-HAART era. The gray line represents the mortality in the HAART era among those who seroconverted before the introduction of HAART, dark gray line represents the mortality among those who seroconverted after HAART. *Source*: Taken from Ref. 64.

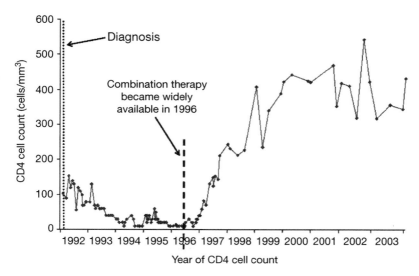

Figure 2 CD4 cell counts measured pre-HAART and in HAART era. Health Protection Agency. *Source*: Taken from Ref. 65.

show a significant rise in CD4 cell counts since the introduction of HAART in 1996 (Fig. 2). HAART uses a combination of powerful drugs, defined as at least triple therapy including two nucleoside reverse transcriptase inhibitors (NRTIs) plus at least one protease inhibitor (PI) or one nonnucleoside reverse transcriptase inhibitor (NNRTI) or a third NRTI (although very rarely used), to subdue HIV infection and give the body the chance to increase its supply of infection-fighting CD4$^+$ T cells that are destroyed by HIV (66).

HIV in the Elderly in the HAART Era

Old age is associated with an increased mortality rate related to a reduced capacity of the immune system to defend against infection and diseases. The rise in chronic conditions such as heart diseases, diabetes, arthritis, strokes, dementia, and cancer provide further complexities to the treatment strategies. Clinicians are now faced with the prospect of treating the impact of an aging HIV population derived from two sources. In the first, the treatment of HIV/AIDS by HAART has seen a significant rise in life expectancy; this increase in the overall survival rates will present a chronically long-term infected cohort, whose viral load have been effectively controlled through the drug therapy. The impact of chronic infection on the composition and dynamics of the T cells within the immune system will present a number of complex problems. The second cohort will consist of individuals infected later in life who present with advance diseases (i.e., CD4 levels of <200 cells/mm^3) because of the increased likelihood of misdiagnosis due to the similarities with other age-associated diseases and also the perception that older people are not "at risk" from infection (67). The traditional stereotypes of "asexual old age" are changing rapidly as exampled by increased numbers of later-life divorces and remarriage rates; a growing trend for intimate but non-cohabiting relationships among older people (68) and the growing medicalization of sexuality with the aid of medication, such as Viagra®, to improve sexual performance (68). Recent reports have demonstrated a rapid increase in the rates of sexually transmitted diseases in the over 50s with figures showing that 6% of females and 12% of males are being diagnosed with HIV/AIDS (68). Other studies have reported as high as 20% of the HIV-positive population being over the age of 50 years (69) (Fig. 3).

Studies examining the impact of HAART on the incidences and causes of death (COD) have noted a significant decline in the AIDS-defining events since its introduction in 1996. Typically AIDS-defining events include non-Hodgkin lymphoma, Cytomegalovirus disease, tuberculosis, *Pneumocystis jiroveci* pneumonia, *Mycobacterium avium* intracellular disseminated infection, progressive multifocal leucoencephalopathy, toxoplasmic encephalitis, disseminated cryptococcosis and Kaposi sarcoma. In the study by Martinez et al. (66), COD in patients diagnosed between January 1997 and December 2004, in Spain, were

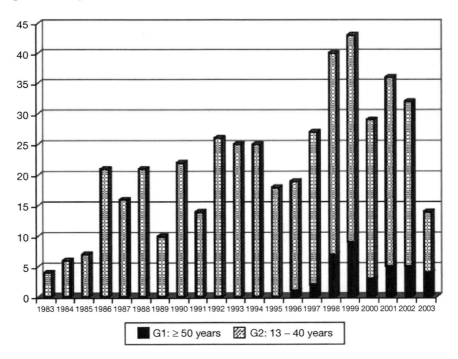

Figure 3 Evolution of HIV diagnosed cases according to age groups. *Source*: Taken from Ref. 95.

shown to experience a yearly decrease of AID-defining events from 84% in 1997 to 7% in 2004. By comparison in the Non-AIDS-defining events, including late-stage liver diseases (hepatitis B and C virus related), nonviral cirrhosis, neoplasia of lung and colon, cardiovascular disease, myocardial infarction, and cerebrovascular disease. An increased incidence from 6% to 44% has been observed. Furthermore, multivariate analysis indicated that CD4 cell counts of less than 200 cells/μL, at the time of HAART initiation and/or increasing plasma viral load, were identified as independent risk factors of dying from an AIDS-defining event. Interestingly, the study highlighted substantial changes in the COD, with cardiovascular disease and late-stage liver disease accounting for approximately 10% and 40% of deaths, respectively (66).

In a similar study, Palella et al. (70) reported a decline in registered deaths from 7 deaths per 100 person-years in 1996 to 1.3 deaths per 100 person-years in 2004 patients, while noting that HAART utilization rates rose from 43% to 82% over the same period. The major findings of this study were the same as those reported by Martinez et al., however, in addition Palella et al. highlighted a substantial proportion of the death by hepatic diseases also reported coinfection with hepatitis B and C viruses, which had risen from 50% in 1996 to 80% in 2004. A noteworthy observation by Palella et al. showed that at the time of death only 40% of AIDS-defining events were receiving HAART compared with 52% of those in non-AIDS-defining events with median ages of 39 and 49 years, respectively. Both patient cohorts described were aged between 16 and 64 years (70). These studies echoed the findings of Lewden et al. (71) in the French population, however COD comparison made between HIV/AIDS individuals and the general population revealed that with increasing age the major COD closely mirrored that of the general population. In subjects below 45 years, infections were the predominant COD whereas above 45 years the leading COD were tumors and cardiovascular diseases (Fig. 4) (71).

HAART and the Elderly

In the pre-HAART era, advanced age was described as a risk factor for progressive HIV disease and increased morbidity and mortality (72). Since the introduction of HAART, limited data is available on antiretroviral therapy in the elderly with very few studies including individuals over the age of 65 years (73). As diagnosis of many older individual occurs at a more advanced disease stage, this represents a more unfavorable prognosis, due to blunted immune reconstitution, more frequent and severe untoward events and more severe short- and long-term drug toxicity (74).

Nevertheless, the limited studies examining the effects of HAART in the over 50s have provided evidence to suggest that advanced age does not seem to affect drug-related toxicity and adherence (67,75). An extensive review of clinical management of HIV in elderly can be found elsewhere (74). One could argue that with changes in social behaviors of the older generation coupled to the

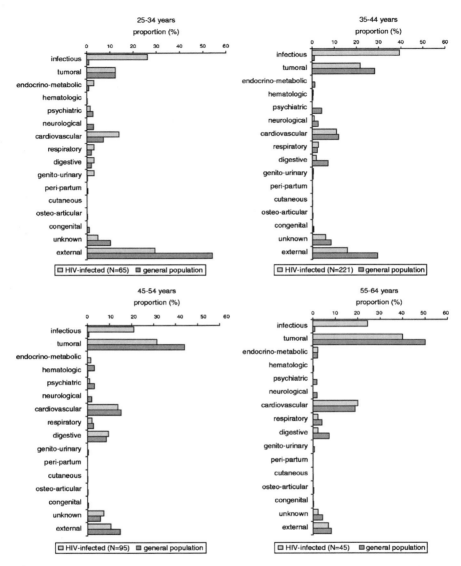

Figure 4 Distribution of the underlying causes of non-HIV-related deaths in 426 HIV-infected adults aged 25 to 64 years (France, 2000) compared with the distribution of the causes of death in the general population (France, 1999). *Source*: Taken from Ref. 71.

success of the HAART drug regime that over the next decade there will be a significant increase in the number of individuals living with HIV in later life.

This may well be reflected in the COD. Historically, the most predominant COD in HIV individuals was opportunistic infections, whereas COD in the general population over 65 years is circulatory disease, followed by respiratory diseases and cancers. As demonstrated in the Lewden study, with increasing age there has been a transition from traditional HIV-related illness such as infection to diseases that more closely resemble those of the general population (Fig. 4). Several studies have reported on the increased likelihood of developing disorders, such as HIV/AIDS-associated dementia (HAD), which has been shown to be 3.26 times more likely in elderly HIV/AIDS patients compared with younger cohorts (69,76); CMV disease has a 5 times higher rate; and Karposi sarcoma 2.3 times higher rate (77).

One final consideration is the impact that comorbidities associated with old age, i.e., diabetes mellitus and malignancies, may interact with the HAART; in particular, the potential toxic or adverse effects that may result from multidrug regimes. Studies investigating renal and hepatic function have demonstrated reduction in both organs in older individuals (78). This may result higher serum levels of HIV drugs and decreased tolerability (79). Furthermore, the range of different HAART drugs possesses the potential for adverse event. Knobel demonstrated that only 36% of those over the age of 60 years continued using a regimen containing PI inhibitor for 2 years compared with 65% in the younger individuals (80). Evidence shows that HIV-infected individuals are at higher risk of cardiovascular disease and metabolic complication that significantly rises based on age and duration of HAART exposure (81). These findings suggest that careful consideration and investigation of HAART drug combination and its potential toxicities are required for effective management of the treatment in later life.

The Paradox of HIV/AIDS and Aging

Despite the advances in our scientific understanding and therapeutic approaches, which allow us to discuss the associations of HIV in the context of an aging population, the stark reality for approximately two-thirds of infected individuals is that they will experience severe reduction in life expectancy. In 2002, the UNAIDS report estimated that HIV/AIDS claimed 3.1 million lives and has been predicted to account for a further 68 million deaths in the 45 most affected countries in the 20 years between 2000 and 2020. The forecasted death toll is greatest in sub-Saharan Africa, where in the 20-year period, 2000 to 2020, 55 million HIV-related deaths are predicted. HIV/AIDS is decreasing the life expectancy in sub-Saharan Africa where the average life expectancy is 47 years, without HIV/AIDS this would have been 62 years. In Botswana, which has the highest adult HIV infection rate (38.8%), the life expectancy at birth had fallen to below 40 years, the lowest seen in Botswana, since the 1950s (82). In the latest United Nations report in 2007, the life expectancy in Botswana has increased from 39 to 47 years following the introduction of 90% treatment coverage (83). At this current rate, by 2050 the average life expectancy is predicted to be 62 years, suggesting that with effective treatment and education programs, there will be a realistic prospect for discussing HIV/AIDS and aging as a global issue.

KEY POINTS

- In developed countries the average life expectancy is 67 years, which is predicted to continue to increase. One of the consequences of the older population is the concomitant increase in age-related illness and disease. The immune system in the elderly appears to be less effective in combating invading pathogens and therefore renders the elderly more susceptible to infections.
- With changing attitudes to sexuality in the older population but at a same time an ignorance of "at risk behavior", some elderly individuals are at increased risk of being infected with HIV later in life. This adds further complications as any of these individuals are misdiagnosed or present with more advanced disease.
- The ability of HIV/AIDS to infect the organism and overcome the immune defense systems results in the infected individual displaying responses that are similar to those in elderly individuals. Alterations have been seen in a range of immune parameters including CD4:CD8 ratios, production of cytokine-mediated responses, T-cell production, B-cell antibody responses, telomere length, and increased infection rates.
- Prior to the widespread availability of HAART, HIV/AIDS would result in premature death most likely due to opportunistic infections. Since the introduction of HAART, life expectancy has increased for HIV-infected individuals.
- In the HAART era of HIV/AIDS, a larger proportion of HIV-infected elderly individuals will require treatment. HAART regimens have seen a transition from the traditional HIV/AIDS-related illness to illnesses that more closely resemble the uninfected aging general population. Therefore, careful management of these individuals to reduce the adverse effects of interactions between multiple combinations of medication is required.
- By contrast, in the developing world which account for two-thirds of the global HIV/AIDS cases, life expectancy is approximately 47 years well below the established baseline for what is consider old in the developed countries. Thus, there is little need to discuss issues concerning age-related diseases until appropriate measures are introduced to ensure that suitable treatment strategies are available.

CONCLUSION

HIV/AIDS has had and continues to have a profound influence on our understanding of the function of the immune systems. The impact of highly active retroviral therapy has provided a genuine hope of a disease-controlled future to individuals in regions where HAART is available. However, there is a growing realization that accompanying this progress are dynamic changes associated with meeting the challenges posed by both HIV/AIDS and natural aging.

REFERENCES

1. Barre-Sinoussi F, Chermann JC, Rey F, et al. Isolation of a T-lymphotropic retrovirus from a patient at risk for acquired immune deficiency syndrome (AIDS). Science 1983, 220:868–871.
2. Malaguarnera L, Ferlito L, Imbesi RM, et al. Immunosenescence: a review. Arch Gerontol Geriatr 2001; 32:1–14.
3. Pawelec G. Immunosenescence: impact in the young as well as the old? Mech Ageing Dev 1999; 108:1–7.
4. Campisi J. Replicative senescence: an old lives' tale? Cell 1996; 84:497–500.
5. Hirokawa K. Understanding the mechanism of the age-related decline in immune function. Nutr Rev 1992; 50:361–366.
6. Makinodan T, Kay MM. Age influence on the immune system. Adv Immunol 1980; 29:287–330.
7. Garcia-Suarez O, Perez-Perez M, Germana A, et al. Involvement of growth factors in thymic involution. Microsc Res Tech 2003; 62:514–523.
8. Haynes BF, Markert ML, Sempowski GD, et al. The role of the thymus in immune reconstitution in aging, bone marrow transplantation, and HIV-1 infection. Annu Rev Immunol 2000; 18:529–560.
9. George AJ, Ritter MA. Thymic involution with ageing: obsolescence or good housekeeping? Immunol Today 1996; 17:267–272.
10. Steinmann GG. Changes in the human thymus during aging. Curr Top Pathol 1986; 75:43–88.
11. Steinmann GG, Klaus B, Muller-Hermelink HK. The involution of the ageing human thymic epithelium is independent of puberty. A morphometric study. Scand J Immunol 1985; 22:563–575.
12. Aspinall R. Age-associated thymic atrophy in the mouse is due to a deficiency affecting rearrangement of the TCR during intrathymic T cell development. J Immunol 1997; 158:3037–3045.
13. Aspinall R, Andrew D. Thymic involution in aging. J Clin Immunol 2000; 20: 250–256.
14. Fry TJ, Mackall CL. Current concepts of thymic aging. Springer Semin Immunopathol 2002; 24:7–22.
15. Godfrey DI, Kennedy J, Mombaerts P, et al. Onset of TCR-beta gene rearrangement and role of TCR-beta expression during CD3-CD4-CD8- thymocyte differentiation. J Immunol 1994; 152:4783–4792.
16. Godfrey DI, Kennedy J, Suda T, et al. A developmental pathway involving four phenotypically and functionally distinct subsets of CD3-CD4-CD8-triple-negative adult mouse thymocytes defined by CD44 and CD25 expression. J Immunol 1993; 150:4244–4252.
17. Wu L, Scollay R, Egerton M, et al. CD4 expressed on earliest T-lineage precursor cells in the adult murine thymus. Nature 1991; 349:71–74.
18. Shortman K, Wu L. Early T lymphocyte progenitors. Annu Rev Immunol 1996; 14:29–47.
19. Wu L, Li CL, Shortman K. Thymic dendritic cell precursors: relationship to the T lymphocyte lineage and phenotype of the dendritic cell progeny. J Exp Med 1996; 184:903–911.

20. Capone M, Hockett RD Jr., Zlotnik A. Kinetics of T cell receptor beta, gamma, and delta rearrangements during adult thymic development: T cell receptor rearrangements are present in CD44(+)CD25(+) Pro-T thymocytes. Proc Natl Acad Sci U S A 1998; 95:12522–12527.

21. Fehling HJ, von Boehmer H. Early alpha beta T cell development in the thymus of normal and genetically altered mice. Curr Opin Immunol 1997; 9:263–275.

22. Petrie HT, Livak F, Schatz DG, et al. Multiple rearrangements in T cell receptor alpha chain genes maximize the production of useful thymocytes. J Exp Med 1993; 178:615–622.

23. Lerner A, Yamada T, Miller RA. Pgp-1hi T lymphocytes accumulate with age in mice and respond poorly to concanavalin A. Eur J Immunol 1989; 19:977–982.

24. Ernst DN, Hobbs MV, Torbett BE, et al. Differences in the expression profiles of CD45RB, Pgp-1, and 3G11 membrane antigens and in the patterns of lymphokine secretion by splenic CD4+ T cells from young and aged mice. J Immunol 1990; 145:1295–1302.

25. Aquino VM, Douek DC, Berryman B, et al. Evaluation of thymic output by measurement of T-cell-receptor gene rearrangement excisional circles (TREC) in patients who have received fludarabine. Leuk Lymphoma 2003; 44:343–348.

26. Arellano MV, Ordonez A, Ruiz-Mateos E, et al. Thymic function-related markers within the thymus and peripheral blood: are they comparable? J Clin Immunol 2006; 26:96–100.

27. Douek DC, Koup RA. Evidence for thymic function in the elderly. Vaccine 2000; 18:1638–1641.

28. Douek DC, McFarland RD, Keiser PH, et al. Changes in thymic function with age and during the treatment of HIV infection. Nature 1998; 396:690–695.

29. Mitchell WA, Meng I, Nicholson SA, et al. Thymic output, ageing and zinc. Biogerontology 2006; 7:461–470.

30. Pido-Lopez J, Imami N, Aspinall R. Both age and gender affect thymic output: more recent thymic migrants in females than males as they age. Clin Exp Immunol 2001; 125:409–413.

31. Timm JA, Thoman ML. Maturation of CD4+ lymphocytes in the aged microenvironment results in a memory-enriched population. J Immunol 1999; 162: 711–717.

32. MacLennan IC, Toellner KM, Cunningham AF, et al. Extrafollicular antibody responses. Immunol Rev 2003; 194:8–18.

33. Valenzuela HF, Effros RB. Divergent telomerase and CD28 expression patterns in human CD4 and CD8 T cells following repeated encounters with the same antigenic stimulus. Clin Immunol 2002; 105:117–125.

34. Kovaiou RD, Grubeck-Loebenstein B. Age-associated changes within CD4+ T cells. Immunol Lett 2006; 107:8–14.

35. Wikby A, Ferguson F, Forsey R, et al. An immune risk phenotype, cognitive impairment, and survival in very late life: impact of allostatic load in Swedish octogenarian and nonagenarian humans. J Gerontol A Biol Sci Med Sci 2005; 60:556–565.

36. Wikby A, Maxson P, Olsson J, et al. Changes in CD8 and CD4 lymphocyte subsets, T cell proliferation responses and non-survival in the very old: the Swedish longitudinal OCTO-immune study. Mech Ageing Dev 1998; 102:187–198.

37. Rufer N, Brummendorf TH, Kolvraa S, et al. Telomere fluorescence measurements in granulocytes and T lymphocyte subsets point to a high turnover of hematopoietic stem cells and memory T cells in early childhood. J Exp Med 1999; 190:157–167.
38. Gourley TS, Wherry EJ, Masopust D, et al. Generation and maintenance of immunological memory. Semin Immunol 2004; 16:323–333.
39. Kaech SM, Wherry EJ, Ahmed R. Effector and memory T-cell differentiation: implications for vaccine development. Nat Rev Immunol 2002; 2:251–262.
40. Badovinac VP, Messingham KA, Jabbari A, et al. Accelerated CD8+ T-cell memory and prime-boost response after dendritic-cell vaccination. Nat Med 2005; 11: 748–756.
41. Stockinger B, Bourgeois C, Kassiotis G. CD4+ memory T cells: functional differentiation and homeostasis. Immunol Rev 2006; 211:39–48.
42. Sun JC, Williams MA, Bevan MJ. CD4+ T cells are required for the maintenance, not programming, of memory CD8+ T cells after acute infection. Nat Immunol 2004; 5:927–933.
43. Seder RA, Ahmed R. Similarities and differences in CD4+ and CD8+ effector and memory T cell generation. Nat Immunol 2003; 4:835–842.
44. Stevceva L, Yoon V, Anastasiades D, et al. Immune responses to HIV Gp120 that facilitate viral escape. Curr HIV Res 2007; 5:47–54.
45. Imami N, Hardy G, Pires A, et al. Immune reconstitution in HIV-1-infected patients. Curr Opin Investig Drugs 2002; 3:1138–1145.
46. Imami N, Pires A, Hardy G, et al. A balanced type 1/type 2 response is associated with long-term nonprogressive human immunodeficiency virus type 1 infection. J Virol 2002; 76:9011–9023.
47. Wilson JD, Imami N, Watkins A, et al. Loss of CD4+ T cell proliferative ability but not loss of human immunodeficiency virus type 1 specificity equates with progression to disease. J Infect Dis 2000; 182:792–798.
48. Younes SA, Yassine-Diab B, Dumont AR, et al. HIV-1 viremia prevents the establishment of interleukin 2-producing HIV-specific memory CD4+ T cells endowed with proliferative capacity. J Exp Med 2003; 198:1909–1922.
49. Sallusto F, Lenig D, Forster R, et al. Two subsets of memory T lymphocytes with distinct homing potentials and effector functions. Nature 1999; 401:708–712.
50. Harari A, Petitpierre S, Vallelian F, et al. Skewed representation of functionally distinct populations of virus-specific CD4 T cells in HIV-1-infected subjects with progressive disease: changes after antiretroviral therapy. Blood 2004; 103:966–972.
51. Harari A, Vallelian F, Pantaleo G. Phenotypic heterogeneity of antigen-specific CD4 T cells under different conditions of antigen persistence and antigen load. Eur J Immunol 2004; 34:3525–3533.
52. Ameisen JC. Programmed cell death and AIDS: from hypothesis to experiment. Immunol Today 1992; 13:388–391.
53. Mattapallil JJ, Douek DC, Hill B, et al. Massive infection and loss of memory CD4+ T cells in multiple tissues during acute SIV infection. Nature 2005; 434:1093–1097.
54. Appay V, Rowland-Jones SL. Premature ageing of the immune system: the cause of AIDS? Trends Immunol 2002; 23:580–585.
55. Beltz L. Thymic involution and HIV progression. Immunol Today 1999; 20:429.
56. Rosenberg PS, Biggar RJ, Goedert JJ. Declining age at HIV infection in the United States. N Engl J Med 1994; 330:789–790.

57. Appay V, Almeida JR, Sauce D, et al. Accelerated immune senescence and HIV-1 infection. Exp Gerontol 2007; 42:432–437.
58. Kalayjian RC, Landay A, Pollard RB, et al. Age-related immune dysfunction in health and in human immunodeficiency virus (HIV) disease: association of age and HIV infection with naive CD8+ cell depletion, reduced expression of CD28 on CD8+ cells, and reduced thymic volumes. J Infect Dis 2003; 187:1924–1933.
59. Ligthart GJ, Corberand JX, Fournier C, et al. Admission criteria for immunogerontological studies in man: the SENIEUR protocol. Mech Ageing Dev 1984; 28: 47–55.
60. Effros RB, Allsopp R, Chiu CP, et al. Shortened telomeres in the expanded CD28-CD8+ cell subset in HIV disease implicate replicative senescence in HIV pathogenesis. Aids 1996; 10:F17–F22.
61. Brenchley JM, Karandikar NJ, Betts MR, et al. Expression of CD57 defines replicative senescence and antigen-induced apoptotic death of CD8+ T cells. Blood 2003; 101:2711–2720.
62. Day CL, Kaufmann DE, Kiepiela P, et al. PD-1 expression on HIV-specific T cells is associated with T-cell exhaustion and disease progression. Nature 2006; 443: 350–354.
63. Rosignoli G, Cranage A, Burton C, et al. Expression of PD-L1, a marker of disease status, is not reduced by HAART in aviraemic patients. AIDS 2007; 21:1379–1381.
64. Smit C, Geskus R, Walker S, et al. Effective therapy has altered the spectrum of cause-specific mortality following HIV seroconversion. AIDS 2006; 20:741–749.
65. HPA. The national CD4 surveillance scheme. Health Protection Agency. Available at: http://www.hpa.org.uk/infections/topics_az/hiv_and_sti/hiv/epidemiology/cd4. htm. Reviewed November 25, 2004.
66. Martinez E, Milinkovic A, Buira E, et al. Incidence and causes of death in HIV-infected persons receiving highly active antiretroviral therapy compared with estimates for the general population of similar age and from the same geographical area. HIV Med 2007; 8:251–258.
67. Cuzin L, Delpierre C, Gerard S, et al. Immunologic and clinical responses to highly active antiretroviral therapy in patients with HIV infection aged >50 years. Clin Infect Dis 2007; 45:654–657.
68. Gott M. Sexual health and the new ageing. Age Ageing 2006; 35:106–107.
69. Valcour VG, Shikuma CM, Watters MR, et al. Cognitive impairment in older HIV-1-seropositive individuals: prevalence and potential mechanisms. AIDS 2004; 18(suppl 1): S79–S86.
70. Palella FJ Jr., Baker RK, Moorman AC, et al. Mortality in the highly active anti-retroviral therapy era: changing causes of death and disease in the HIV outpatient study. J Acquir Immune Defic Syndr 2006; 43:27–34.
71. Lewden C, Salmon D, Morlat P, et al. Causes of death among human immunodeficiency virus (HIV)-infected adults in the era of potent antiretroviral therapy: emerging role of hepatitis and cancers, persistent role of AIDS. Int J Epidemiol 2005; 34:121–130.
72. Pezzotti P, Phillips AN, Dorrucci M, et al. Category of exposure to HIV and age in the progression to AIDS: longitudinal study of 1199 people with known dates of seroconversion. HIV Italian Seroconversion Study Group. BMJ 1996; 313:583–586.

73. Manfredi R, Calza L, Cocchi D, et al. Antiretroviral treatment and advanced age: epidemiologic, laboratory, and clinical features in the elderly. J Acquir Immune Defic Syndr 2003; 33:112–114.
74. Manfredi R. HIV infection and advanced age emerging epidemiological, clinical, and management issues. Ageing Res Rev 2004; 3:31–54.
75. Sungkanuparph S, Manosuthi W, Kiertiburanakul S, et al. Clinical experience with high success rate of antiretroviral therapy in elderly HIV-infected patients. Age Ageing 2004; 33:520–521.
76. Valcour V, Shikuma C, Shiramizu B, et al. Higher frequency of dementia in older HIV-1 individuals: the Hawaii Aging with HIV-1 Cohort. Neurology 2004; 63: 822–827.
77. Grabar S, Weiss L, Costagliola D. HIV infection in older patients in the HAART era. J Antimicrob Chemother 2006; 57:4–7.
78. Sotaniemi EA, Arranto AJ, Pelkonen O, et al. Age and cytochrome P450-linked drug metabolism in humans: an analysis of 226 subjects with equal histopathologic conditions. Clin Pharmacol Ther 1997; 61:331–339.
79. Casau NC. Perspective on HIV infection and aging: emerging research on the horizon. Clin Infect Dis 2005; 41:855–863.
80. Knobel H, Guelar A, Valldecillo G, et al. Response to highly active antiretroviral therapy in HIV-infected patients aged 60 years or older after 24 months follow-up. AIDS 2001; 15:1591–1593.
81. Friis-Moller N, Sabin CA, Weber R, et al. Combination antiretroviral therapy and the risk of myocardial infarction. N Engl J Med 2003; 349:1993–2003.
82. UNAIDS. Report on the global AIDS epidemic 2002.
83. UN. United Nations, Department of Economic and Social Affairs. World Population Prospects: The 2006 Revision, Highlights, Working Paper No. ESA/P/WP.202, 2007.
84. Prelog M. Aging of the immune system: a risk factor for autoimmunity? Autoimmun Rev 2006; 5:136–139.
85. Gottlieb MS, Schroff R, Schanker HM, et al. Pneumocystis carinii pneumonia and mucosal candidiasis in previously healthy homosexual men: evidence of a new acquired cellular immunodeficiency. N Engl J Med 1981; 305:1425–1431.
86. Hellerstein M, Hanley MB, Cesar D, et al. Directly measured kinetics of circulating T lymphocytes in normal and HIV-1-infected humans. Nat Med 1999; 5:83–89.
87. Pawelec G, Effros RB, Caruso C, et al. T cells and aging (update February 1999). Front Biosci 1999; 4:D216–D269.
88. Fan J, Bass HZ, Fahey JL. Elevated IFN-gamma and decreased IL-2 gene expression are associated with HIV infection. J Immunol 1993; 151:5031–5040.
89. Clerici M, Stocks NI, Zajac RA, et al. Detection of three distinct patterns of T helper cell dysfunction in asymptomatic, human immunodeficiency virus-seropositive patients. Independence of CD4+ cell numbers and clinical staging. J Clin Invest 1989; 84:1892–1899.
90. Franceschi C, Bonafe M, Valensin S. Human immunosenescence: the prevailing of innate immunity, the failing of clonotypic immunity, and the filling of immunological space. Vaccine 2000; 18:1717–1720.
91. Wolthers KC, Bea G, Wisman A, et al. T cell telomere length in HIV-1 infection: no evidence for increased CD4+ T cell turnover. Science 1996; 274:1543–1547.
92. Gougeon ML, Montagnier L. Apoptosis in AIDS. Science 1993; 260:1269–1270.

93. Appay V, Zaunders JJ, Papagno L, et al. Characterization of CD4(+) CTLs ex vivo. J Immunol 2002; 168:5954–5958.
94. Nociari MM, Telford W, Russo C. Postthymic development of CD28-CD8+ T cell subset: age-associated expansion and shift from memory to naive phenotype. J Immunol 1999; 162:3327–3335.
95. Nogueras M, Navarro G, Anton E, et al. Epidemiological and clinical features, response to HAART, and survival in HIV-infected patients diagnosed at the age of 50 or more. BMC Infect Dis 2006; 6:159.
96. Wolthers KC, Otto SA, Lens SM, et al. Increased expression of CD80, CD86 and CD70 on T cells from HIV-infected individuals upon activation in vitro: regulation by CD4+ T cells. Eur J Immunol 1996; 26:1700–1706.
97. Schwartz O, Marechal V, Le Gall S, et al. Endocytosis of major histocompatibility complex class I molecules is induced by the HIV-1 Nef protein. Nat Med 1996; 2:338–342.

2

The Nervous System

Cristian L. Achim and Ian Paul Everall

Department of Psychiatry, University of California,
San Diego, California, U.S.A.

HIV and aging have similar effects on global cognitive functioning. Progressive brain dysfunction associated with aging has been linked to neuronal loss and to physiological impairments with reduced neurotransmitter production and inflammatory processes. This chapter reviews some of the emerging data on central nervous system (CNS) changes associated with HIV disease and aging.

EFFECTS OF AGING ON HIV-ASSOCIATED BRAIN DISEASE

A study published in 2004 (1) found that individuals over 50 years of age represent 11% of the HIV cases registered by the Centers for Disease Control and Prevention (CDC). Twenty percent of the HIV-infected population above the age of 50 years resides in Hawaii. Data from the Hawaii cohort suggest an association between increased neurocognitive impairment in older HIV patients compared with younger controls. Factors leading to this association may include vascular pathology, age-related immunological changes and limited compensatory brain capacity. In a study by Becker and colleagues in Western Pennsylvania (2), the prevalence of cognitive disorder among HIV-positive patients over 50 years was significantly higher than in younger individuals (alcohol abuse was an additional significant risk factor.)

In a cross-sectional study of two groups of patients, either over 50 years old or under 35 years, Cherner and colleagues (3) found that older individuals with detectable virus in the cerebrospinal fluid (CSF) had twice the prevalence of neuropsychological impairment compared with those with undetectable CSF virus. The development of neuropsychological impairment in the younger patients was independent of the CSF viral load. In another study, the authors examined the effect of age and HIV status on 254 individuals. Significant effects for serostatus and age group on overall cognitive abilities were found, after controlling for the effect of education. However, older seropositive individuals were not found to have an increased risk for HIV-related cognitive impairment compared with normal age-related cognitive changes (4).

Tozzi and colleagues (5) analyzed the results of neuropsychological batteries, neuromedical examinations, and brain imaging in a study of 94 patients on HAART and found that persistent neuropsychological deficits were observed in 63% of the patients and that the only significant correlate (vs. age, gender, CDC stage, CD4 count, and viral load) was the severity of neurocognitive impairment (NCI) at the start of HAART initiation. These results indicate that HAART should be started immediately when NCI is recognized.

Goodkin highlighted the importance of psychiatric diseases in the aging HIV-infected population (6). In a study of prevalence rates of major depressive disorder and substance use disorders, Rabkin and colleagues (7) found that while the rates of these disorders declined with age in an HIV-uninfected cohort, the rates of major depression and substance use remained persistently high in aging HIV-infected individuals. Another study of aging veterans noted similar high rates of major depression and substance use, which declined with age in the HIV-uninfected but not in the HIV-infected group (8). In this study, memory problems were associated with aging in both groups. It is possible that enhanced survival with chronic HIV brain infection results in a spectrum of damage. Neurocognitive impairment and major depressive disorder have similarities in terms of neuropsychological, neuroimaging, and neuropathological findings. Depression is associated with decreased levels of the neurotransmitter dopamine. Major depression in the setting of HIV has been associated with significant loss in the gene expression for somatostatin, which is thought to modulate dopamine levels (9).

MECHANISMS OF BRAIN DISEASE

HAART has changed the patterns of HIV-related neuropathology and clinical manifestations in the past 10 years with the emergence of new variants of HIV encephalopathy, including white matter injury, "burnt-out" pathology, and amyloid deposition (10). Factors contributing to this new spectrum of pathologies include viral resistance to HAART, immune reconstitution, HAART neurotoxicity, and comorbid factors like methamphetamine and hepatitis C virus (HCV). A paramount copathogenic factor in the long-term surviving patients with HIV on HAART is age.

The factors modulating brain disease may be local (organ specific) or systemic (e.g., metabolic, vascular, or inflammatory). For example, in the

Hawaii aging cohort, neurocognitive impairment was associated with diabetes; this finding was not explained by age, vascular risk factors, or the HIV/ HAART status (11). Insulin resistance is associated with lower cognitive performance in the HIV-infected patients enrolled in the Hawaii aging cohort, suggesting that metabolic dysfunction may contribute to neuropathogenesis in the HAART era (12). ApoE genotype was determined for 182 participants in the Hawaii aging cohort and an independent (after controlling for age or diabetes) risk of neurocognitive impairment related to ApoE4 was seen in older subjects (13).

Normal aging and HIV infection may lead to inflammatory changes in the brain, but the mechanisms are not clear. By using proton magnetic resonance spectroscopy (H-MRS) in a study of 46 HIV patients naïve to antiretroviral therapy, it was found that compared with controls, there was neuronal damage in the basal ganglia and glial cell activation in the frontal white matter beyond that observed in normal aging (14). Another MRS study of the brain in aging HIV-infected patients found that glial cell activation is probably initiated during the neuroasymptomatic (NAS) stages and that continued inflammatory activity and neuronal injury in the basal ganglia and white matter are associated with the development of neurocognitive impairment (15). Furthermore, by using contrast-enhanced magnetic resonance imaging (CE-MRI), Avison et al. found that the severity of neurocognitive impairment correlates with the degree of blood brain barrier breakdown in the basal ganglia and that HAART may have a protective effect (16).

The consensus among neuropathologists, on the basis of a large number of autopsy studies, is that the brain macrophages are the main host and carriers of the virus into the brain (17–23). Macrophage-associated neurtoxins studied in conjunction with HIV include a spectrum of monokines, chemokines, other mediators of inflammation, viral proteins, nitric oxide, and some still unidentified factors (24,25). The origins of these HIV-infected macrophages (parenchymal vs. vascular) differs in various experimental models (26,27). However, there is little debate on the central role played by brain macrophages and microglia in the pathogenesis of neurocognitive impairment in HIV infection, as was recently highlighted in a comprehensive review by Gonzales-Scarano and Martin-Garcia (28).

BETA-AMYLOID DEPOSITION

Previous studies of beta-amyloid (β-amyloid) deposition in the HIV brain have focused on the human β-amyloid precursor protein (APP), which is considered by many to be a marker of neuronal degeneration. Several reports have described a significant increase in brain APP in AIDS, specifically in the axons of the subcortical white matter tracts.

One leading theory is based on the inflammatory response in HIV infection of the brain parenchyma, where activated microglia are considered by many to be the likely source of mediators of disease that can promote over-production and accumulation of APP (29,30). Among the brain macrophage–secreted factors mediating the overproduction of neuronal APP, a leading candidate is IL-1 (31).

The association between the brain pathology characteristic of HIV encephalopathy, including viral proteins and the presence of APP aggregates, often as intra-axonal globules, was reported in several studies (32–34) . In general, these studies have shown overproduction and intra-axonal accumulation of APP to be not only a marker of neuronal degeneration but also a mediator of it.

The majority of the studies show a strong correlation between the topography of HIV-associated pathology and degenerating axons, suggesting a local, intraparenchymal effect on APP accumulation. However, at least one study of APP in the HIV brain, Scaravilli and colleagues (35) did not find a good correlation between APP and microgliosis and concluded that the axonal degeneration in HIV infection may be due to systemic factors (e.g., cytokines).

Several studies showed that APP deposition may precede β-amyloid accumulation (36) in the vicinity of synapses, suggesting that APP may be processed at these sites. Other investigators believe that β-amyloid deposition is the primary event that, in combination with the surrounding reactive glia, may lead to APP accumulation in degenerating neurites (37). In vitro, β-amyloid treatments induce degeneration of neurites similar to Alzheimer's disease (38), possibly by inhibiting fast axonal anterograde transport (39).

The ongoing clinical studies of β-amyloid and tau in the CSF have generated some controversial results, often because of the differences in the methodology used. While β-amyloid levels may be both up- and downregulated in the CSF of HIV patients, there is a consensus building toward interpreting increased levels of hyperphosphorylated tau as an indicator or neuronal pathology that may be associated with neurocognitive impairment in HIV (40–43).

IMPACT OF HAART

In the era of efficient antiviral therapies, there seems to be a significant decrease in the severity of neurological symptoms in HIV-infected patients (44,45). The cohort studies evaluating the efficacy of HAART or even less aggressive treatments (e.g., AZT) in preventing neurological disease have found that increased survival on treatment is most often accompanied by reduced HIV-associated brain pathology. (29,46–51). The strongest evidence was published by Vago et al. (52), who reported an almost fourfold decrease in the prevalence of HIV-related CNS pathology in the patients on HAART compared with those from the pre-AZT era. Nonetheless, another large cohort retrospective study from Europe showed that even in patients responding to HAART, the brain is still the second most frequently involved organ (after the lung) (53).

In a 2006 review, Valcour and Paul discuss the impact of aging on HIV-associated neurocognitive impairment and the benefit of adjunctive therapies

(54). Older patients were previously thought to have a higher risk of HIV-associated dementia. But a recent study demonstrates that this pattern may have changed in the HAART era. Larussa and colleagues (55) have shown that in a cohort of 195 patients, half diagnosed with dementia and half with minor cognitive motor disorder (MCMD), older age was associated with dementia, but only in the patients without antiviral therapy. Furthermore, there was no significant effect of age in the patients with MCMD on HAART, suggesting that the antiviral therapy may have a neuroprotective effect in older patients. Another study showed white matter disease (by MRI) in aging patients in the HAART era may be related more to small vessel–associated ischemia than HIV (56).

HAART has been available for most HIV patients in France since 1996. From a survey of 343 brains from AIDS patients who died between 1985 and 2002, it was found that despite a dramatic decrease in the number of autopsies, brain involvement remained a major cause of death (57); this study series found the emergence of a new variant of HIV encephalopathy: severe leukoencephalopathy with mononuclear infiltration, possibly due to the response from the newly reconstituted immune system. In a series of autopsy studies from patients who died with HIV but failed HAART, Langford and colleagues (58) found a changing pattern of pathology, marked predominantly by demyelination and inflammatory infiltrates.

While the clinical benefit in reducing viral burden is indisputable, HAART is also reported to induce metabolic dysregulation resulting in a syndrome of lipodystrophy (LD) in up to 83% of treated individuals (59). Features associated with LD include insulin resistance with hyperinsulinemia, centripetal lipohypertrophy with concurrent subcutaneous peripheral lipoatrophy, and hypertriglyceridemia.

The metabolic complications underlying LD include insulin resistance. Insulin protease, or insulin degradation enzyme (IDE), insulinase, or insulysin, is a zinc-binding metalloprotease of the peptidase family M16, located on chromosome 10. The main function of IDE appears to be the degradation of insulin, but it is also the key enzyme in the degradation of β-amyloid as well as other substrates such as transforming growth factor alpha (TGF-α). The protein degradation functions of IDE are complemented by additional activities, such as proteolytic processing of β endorphin and regulation of androgen and glucocorticoid receptors. Although ubiquitously expressed (60), the major function of IDE in the brain is to break down amyloid (61). Competitive inhibition of amyloid degradation by insulin has been demonstrated in vitro (61). Other studies have demonstrated a genetic linkage with Alzheimer's disease and chromosome 10q (62), the locus of the IDE gene.

A recently completed autopsy study from Scotland (63) showed that in the post-HAART era the levels of microglial activation in two key regions of the brain, the basal ganglia and hippocampus, were actually higher compared with pre-HAART controls, suggesting that there is a surprising degree of ongoing neuroinflammation in these patients, which may be of concern in the long term and pathologically relevant to the aging population.

CONCLUSION

There is a growing recognition that although the introduction of HAART has revolutionized the prognosis of people living with HIV, this population now faces new challenges with aging. There appears to be evidence for accelerated aging with increased risks of developing neurocognitive impairment due to a multitude of factors. As summarized in Figure 1, they include the following: drugs abuse, which is associated with exacerbating cognitive performance in the setting of HIV; HIV itself, including the emerging drug-resistant strains whose effect is not yet apparent; host responses, including CD4 recovery, inheritance of ApoE4, and other immune indicators; and the effect of antiretrovirals, which can result in metabolic complications including insulin resistance. Insulin resistance can accelerate amyloid and hyperphosphorylated tau deposition, thereby enhancing the risk of other common neurodegenerative disorders such as Alzheimer's disease, while other metabolic complications in the setting of aging can elevate the risk of vascular disorders such as microinfarcts or stroke.

Questions regarding the impact of HAART and aging on HIV-associated CNS disease progression will be answered more thoroughly by several ongoing longitudinal studies. Some of these cohorts have been assembled by the HIV Neurobehavioral Research Center (HNRC) at University of California, San Diego, the Veterans Aging Cohort Study (VACS), and the Hawaii aging cohort. VACS is well positioned to study HIV as a chronic disease in the aging population (64); the goal is to analyze the influence of age and mediating factors on outcomes with HIV. Veterans with HIV infection have characteristics that will

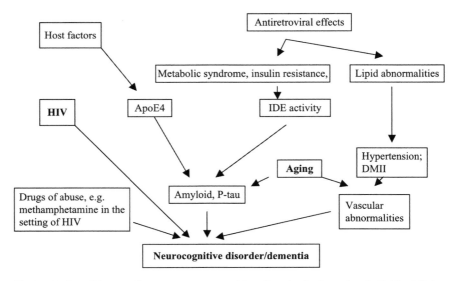

Figure 1 Possible contributors to neurocognitive disorder in the aging individual living with HIV.

likely become more prevalent in the Unite States: they are older, commonly suffer comorbid disease, and are often members of minority populations (65).

Although HAART is essential and effective, it may be necessary in the long term to provide additional neuroprotection. Indications are that infection is not completely eradicated and neurotoxicity may continue despite HAART (66). Furthermore, chronic care in older HIV patients may require diligence to diagnose and treat other CNS pathologies associated with aging, such as Alzheimer's disease (67).

REFERENCES

1. Valcour V, Shikuma C, Shiramizu B, et al. Higher frequency of dementia in older HIV-1 individuals: the Hawaii Aging with HIV-1 Cohort. Neurology 2004; 63(5): 822–827.
2. Becker JT, Lopez OL, Dew MA, et al. Prevalence of cognitive disorders differs as a function of age in HIV virus infection. AIDS 2004; 18(suppl 1):S11–S18.
3. Cherner M, Ellis RJ, Lazzaretto D, et al. Effects of HIV-1 infection and aging on neurobehavioral functioning: preliminary findings. AIDS 2004; 18(suppl 1): S27–S34.
4. Kissel EC, Pukay-Martin ND, Bornstein RA. The relationship between age and cognitive function in HIV-infected men. J Neuropsychiatry Clin Neurosci 2005; 17(2): 180–184.
5. Tozzi V, Balestra P, Balestra P, et al. Persistence of neuropsychologic deficits despite long-term highly active antiretroviral therapy in patients with HIV-related neurocognitive impairment: prevalence and risk factors. J Acquir Immune Defic Syndr 2007; 45(2):174–182.
6. Goodkin K, Wilkie FL, Concha M, et al. Aging and neuro-AIDS conditions and the changing spectrum of HIV-1-associated morbidity and mortality. J Clin Epidemiol 2001; 54(suppl 1):S35–S43.
7. Rabkin JG, McElhiney MC, Ferrando SJ. Mood and substance use disorders in older adults with HIV/AIDS: methodological issues and preliminary evidence. AIDS 2004; 18(suppl 1):S43–S48.
8. Justice AC, McGinnis KA, Atkinson JH, et al. Veterans Aging Cohort 5-Site Study Project Team. Psychiatric and neurocognitive disorders among HIV-positive and negative veterans in care: Veterans Aging Cohort Five-Site Study. AIDS 2004; 18 (suppl 1): S49–S59.
9. Everall IP, Salaria S, Atkinson JH, et al. HNRC (HIV Neurobehavioral Research Center). Diminished somatostatin gene expression in individuals with HIV and major depressive disorder. Neurology 2006; 67(10):1867–1869.
10. Everall IP, Hansen LA, Masliah E. The shifting patterns of HIV encephalitis neuropathology. Neurotox Res 2005; 8(1–2):51–61.
11. Valcour VG, Shikuma CM, Shiramizu BT, et al. Diabetes, insulin resistance, and dementia among HIV-1-infected patients. J Acquir Immune Defic Syndr 2005; 38(1): 31–36.
12. Valcour VG, Sacktor NC, Paul RH, et al. Insulin resistance is associated with cognition among HIV-1-infected patients: the Hawaii Aging With HIV cohort. J Acquir Immune Defic Syndr 2006; 43(4):405–410.

13. Valcour V, Shikuma C, Shiramizu B, et al. Age, apolipoprotein E4, and the risk of HIV dementia: the Hawaii Aging with HIV Cohort. J Neuroimmunol 2004; 157(1–2):197–202.
14. Ernst T, Chang L. Effect of aging on brain metabolism in antiretroviral-naive HIV patients. AIDS 2004; 18(suppl 1):S61–S67.
15. Chang L, Lee PL, Yiannoutsos CT, et al. A multicenter in vivo proton-MRS study of HIV-associated dementia and its relationship to age. Neuroimage 2004; 23(4): 1336–1347.
16. Avison MJ, Nath A, Greene-Avison R, et al. Neuroimaging correlates of HIV-associated BBB compromise. J Neuroimmunol 2004; 157(1–2):140–146.
17. Epstein LG, Sharer LR, Cho ES, et al. HTLV-III/LAV-like retrovirus particles in the brains of patients with AIDS encephalopathy. AIDS Res 1984; 1:447–454.
18. Petito CK, Navia BA, Cho ES, et al. Vacuolar myelopathy pathologically resembling subacute combined degeneration in patients with the acquired immunodeficiency syndrome. N Engl J Med 1985; 312:874–879.
19. Shaw GM, Harper ME, Hahn BH, et al. HTLV-III infection in brains of children and adults with AIDS encephalopathy. Science 1985; 227:177–182.
20. Navia BA, Cho ES, Petito CK, et al. The AIDS dementia complex: II. Neuropathology. Ann Neurol 1986; 19:525–535.
21. Navia BA, Jordan BD, Price RW. The AIDS dementia complex: I. Clinical features. Ann Neurol 1986; 19:517–524.
22. Petito CK, Cho ES, Lemann W, et al. Neuropathology of acquired immunodeficiency syndrome (AIDS): an autopsy review. J Neuropathol Exp Neurol 1986; 45(6):635–646.
23. Wiley C, Schrier RD, Nelson JA, et al. Cellular localization of human immunodeficiency virus infection within the brains of acquired immune deficiency syndrome patients. Proc Natl Acad Sci USA 1986; 83:7089–7093.
24. Brana C, Biggs TE, Barton CH, et al. A soluble factor produced by macrophages mediates the neurotoxic effects of HIV-1 Tat in vitro. AIDS 1999; 13(12):1443–1452.
25. Xiong H, Zeng YC, Zheng J, et al. Soluble HIV-1 infected macrophage secretory products mediate blockade of long-term potentiation: a mechanism for cognitive dysfunction in HIV-1-associated dementia [In Process Citation]. J Neurovirol 1999; 5(5):519–528.
26. Williams KC, Corey S, Westmoreland SV, et al. Perivascular macrophages are the primary cell type productively infected by simian immunodeficiency virus in the brains of macaques: implications for the neuropathogenesis of AIDS. J Exp Med 2001; 193(8):905–915.
27. Cosenza MA, Zhao ML, Si Q, et al. Human brain parenchymal microglia express CD14 and CD45 and are productively infected by HIV-1 in HIV-1 encephalitis. Brain Pathol 2002; 12(4):442–455.
28. Gonzalez-Scarano F, Martin-Garcia J. The neuropathogenesis of AIDS. Nat Rev Immunol 2005; 5(1):69–81.
29. Adle-Biassette H, Chretien F, Wingertsmann L, et al. Neuronal apoptosis does not correlate with dementia in HIV infection but is related to microglial activation and axonal damage. Neuropathol Appl Neurobiol 1999; 25(2):123–133.
30. Dickson DW, Lee SC, Mattiace LA, et al. Microglia and cytokines in neurological disease, with special reference to AIDS and Alzheimer's disease. Glia 1993; 7(1):75–83.
31. Stanley LC, Mrak RE, Woody RC, et al. Glial cytokines as neuropathogenic factors in HIV infection: pathogenic similarities to Alzheimer's disease. J Neuropathol Exp Neurol 1994; 53(3):231–238.

32. Giometto B, An SF, Groves M, et al. Accumulation of beta-amyloid precursor protein in HIV encephalitis: relationship with neuropsychological abnormalities. Ann Neurol 1997; 42(1):34–40.
33. Raja F, Sherriff FE, Morris CS, et al. Cerebral white matter damage in HIV infection demonstrated using beta-amyloid precursor protein immunoreactivity. Acta Neuropathol (Berl) 1997; 93(2):184–189.
34. Nebuloni M, Pellegrinelli A, Ferri A, et al. Beta amyloid precursor protein and patterns of HIV p24 immunohistochemistry in different brain areas of AIDS patients. AIDS 2001; 15(5):571–575.
35. An SF, Giometto B, Groves M, et al. Axonal damage revealed by accumulation of beta-APP in HIV-positive individuals without AIDS. J Neuropathol Exp Neurol 1997; 56(11):1262–1268.
36. Ichihara N, Wu J, Chui DH, et al. Axonal degeneration promotes abnormal accumulation of amyloid beta-protein in ascending gracile tract of gracile axonal dystrophy (GAD) mouse. Brain Res 1995; 695(2):173–178.
37. Ohgami T, Kitamoto T, Weidmann A, et al. Alzheimer's amyloid precursor protein-positive degenerative neurites exist even within kuru plaques not specific to Alzheimer's disease. Am J Pathol 1991; 139(6):1245–1250.
38. Pike CJ, Cummings BJ, Cotman CW. Beta-Amyloid induces neuritic dystrophy in vitro: similarities with Alzheimer pathology. Neuroreport 1992; 3(9):769–772.
39. Kasa P, Papp H, Kovacs I, et al. Human amyloid-beta1-42 applied in vivo inhibits the fast axonal transport of proteins in the sciatic nerve of rat. Neurosci Lett 2000; 278(1–2):117–119.
40. Andersson L, Blennow K, Fuchs D, et al. Increased cerebrospinal fluid protein tau concentration in neuro-AIDS. J Neurol Sci 1999; 171(2):92–96.
41. Brew BJ, Pemberton L, Blennow K, et al. CSF amyloid beta42 and tau levels correlate with AIDS dementia complex. Neurology 2005; 65(9):1490–1492.
42. Andersson LM, Hagberg L, Rosengren L, et al. Normalisation of cerebrospinal fluid biomarkers parallels improvement of neurological symptoms following HAART in HIV dementia—case report. BMC Infect Dis 2006; 6:141.
43. Fellgiebel A, Scheurich A, Bartenstein P, et al. FDG-PET and CSF phospho-tau for prediction of cognitive decline in mild cognitive impairment. Psychiatry Res 2007; 155(2):167–171.
44. Price RW, Yiannoutsos CT, Clifford DB, et al. Neurological outcomes in late HIV infection: adverse impact of neurological impairment on survival and protective effect of antiviral therapy. AIDS Clinical Trial Group and Neurological AIDS Research Consortium study team. AIDS 1999; 13(13):1677–1685.
45. Tozzi V, Balestra P, Galgani S, et al. Positive and sustained effects of highly active antiretroviral therapy on HIV-1-associated neurocognitive impairment [In Process Citation]. AIDS 1999; 13(14):1889–1897.
46. Baldeweg T, Catalan J, Gazzard BG. Risk of HIV dementia and opportunistic brain disease in AIDS and zidovudine therapy. J Neurol Neurosurg Psychiatry 1998; 65(1): 34–41.
47. Chang L, Ernst T, Leonido-Yee M, et al. Highly active antiretroviral therapy reverses brain metabolite abnormalities in mild HIV dementia. Neurology 1999; 53(4):782–789.
48. Gavin P, Yogev R. Central nervous system abnormalities in pediatric human immunodeficiency virus infection. Pediatr Neurosurg 1999; 31(3):115–123.

49. Pezzotti P, Serraino D, Rezza G, et al. The spectrum of AIDS-defining diseases: temporal trends in Italy prior to the use of highly active anti-retroviral therapies, 1982–1996. Int J Epidemiol 1999; 28(5):975–981.
50. Raskino C, Pearson DA, Baker CJ, et al. Neurologic, neurocognitive, and brain growth outcomes in human immunodeficiency virus-infected children receiving different nucleoside antiretroviral regimens. Pediatric AIDS Clinical Trials Group 152 Study Team. Pediatrics 1999; 104(3):e32.
51. von Giesen HJ, Hefter H, Jablonowski H, et al. HAART is neuroprophylactic in HIV-1 infection. J Acquir Immune Defic Syndr 2000; 23(5):380–385.
52. Vago L, Bonetto S, Nebuloni M, et al. Pathological findings in the central nervous system of AIDS patients on assumed antiretroviral therapeutic regimens: retrospective study of 1597 autopsies. AIDS 2002; 16(14):1925–1928.
53. Jellinger KA, Setinek U, Drlicek M, et al. Neuropathology and general autopsy findings in AIDS during the last 15 years. Acta Neuropathol (Berl) 2000; 100(2): 213–220.
54. Valcour V, Paul R. HIV infection and dementia in older adults. Clin Infect Dis 2006; 42(10):1449–1454.
55. Larussa D, Lorenzini P, Cingolani A, et al. Highly active antiretroviral therapy reduces the age-associated risk of dementia in a cohort of older HIV-1-infected patients. AIDS Res Hum Retroviruses 2006; 22(5):386–392.
56. McMurtray A, Nakamoto B, Shikuma C, et al. Small-vessel vascular disease in human immunodeficiency virus Infection: the Hawaii Aging with HIV Cohort Study. Cerebrovasc Dis 2007; 24(2–3):236–241.
57. Gray F, Chrétien F, Vallat-Decouvelaere AV, et al. The changing pattern of HIV neuropathology in the HAART era. J Neuropathol Exp Neurol 2003; 62(5):429–440.
58. Langford TD, Letendre SL, Marcotte TD, et al. Severe, demyelinating leukoencephalopathy in AIDS patients on antiretroviral therapy. AIDS 2002; 16(7):1019–1029.
59. Carr A, Samaras K, Thorisdottir A, et al. Diagnosis, prediction, and natural course of HIV-1 protease-inhibitor-associated lipodystrophy, hyperlipidaemia, and diabetes mellitus: a cohort study. Lancet 1999; 353(9170):2093–2099.
60. Kuo WL, Montag AG, Rosner MR. Insulin-degrading enzyme is differentially expressed and developmentally regulated in various rat tissues. Endocrinology 1993; 132(2):604–611.
61. Qiu WQ, Walsh DM, Ye Z, et al. Insulin-degrading enzyme regulates extracellular levels of amyloid beta-protein by degradation. J Biol Chem 1998; 273(49): 32730–32738.
62. Bertram L, Blacker D, Mullin K, et al. Evidence for genetic linkage of Alzheimer's disease to chromosome 10q. Science 2000; 290(5500):2302–2303.
63. Anthony IC, Ramage SN, Carnie FW, et al. Influence of HAART on HIV-related CNS disease and neuroinflammation. J Neuropathol Exp Neurol 2005; 64(6):529–536.
64. Justice AC, Landefeld CS, Asch SM, et al. Justification for a new cohort study of people aging with and without HIV infection. J Clin Epidemiol 2001; 54(suppl 1): S3–S8.
65. Smola S, Justice AC, Wagner J, et al. Veterans aging cohort three-site study (VACS 3): overview and description. J Clin Epidemiol 2001; 54(suppl 1):S61–S76.
66. Clifford DB. AIDS dementia. Med Clin North Am 2002; 86(3):537–550, vi.
67. Alisky JM. The coming problem of HIV-associated Alzheimer's disease. Med Hypotheses 2007.

3

Depression

Edward R. Hammond

*Departments of Psychiatry and Neurology, Johns Hopkins
University School of Medicine, Baltimore, Maryland, U.S.A.*

Glenn J. Treisman

*Departments of Psychiatry, Behavioral Sciences and Internal Medicine,
Johns Hopkins University School of Medicine, Baltimore, Maryland, U.S.A.*

INTRODUCTION

Patients with HIV are living longer because of the remarkable strides that have been made in understanding and treating both the virus and the complications associated with it. Psychiatry has become increasingly important to HIV care providers because of the high rates of psychiatric comorbidity found in HIV populations. Psychiatric disorders not only play a role in the behaviors that get people infected but also have a profound influence on heath care access and adherence to medical recommendations. Unfortunately, not much research has been done in the area of geriatric HIV psychiatry, but there is some useful information from the geriatric psychiatry literature that bears directly on treating patients with HIV, and psychiatric studies in younger patients with HIV that are applicable to elderly HIV-infected patients. The "elderly" among the HIV population typically refer to those living with HIV over the age of 50 years. Data from the Centers for Disease Control and Prevention (CDC) indicate that between the years 2001 and 2005, the estimated number of persons living with

HIV in 33 states and U.S.-dependent areas with confidential name-based HIV reporting increased by 77% (1). At the end of 2005, 24.4% of people living with HIV were above the age of 50 years, an increase from 16.8% in 2001 (1). The elderly HIV patients consist of two populations, the long-term HIV survivors and older adults who are newly infected. The time to diagnose HIV in the elderly has been shown to be delayed (2). In the elderly, initial symptoms of fatigue, weight loss, shortness of breath, and poor memory may be mistakenly attributed to the aging process. Prevention efforts generally have not included the elderly in efforts to increase safe sex practices (condom use), and there is less of an issue of pregnancy in this population, and finally, many of these patients developed their sexual practices in the pre-HIV era, leading to risky behavior. This coupled with inadequate supporting structures increases the risk of HIV acquisition in the elderly (3).

In addition to efforts aimed at preventing HIV infection in the elderly, there needs to be a whole patient approach to the care of the elderly that includes integrated treatment for those who are presently living with HIV. Psychiatric comorbidity, medical issues associated with aging, and loss of social foundation related to retirement, death of partners, and dispersion of family are of importance in this approach. The presence of HIV/AIDS increases the lifetime prevalence of psychiatric diagnosis, while the presence of psychiatric disorder increases the risk of HIV infection (4). Figure 1 is a conceptual framework

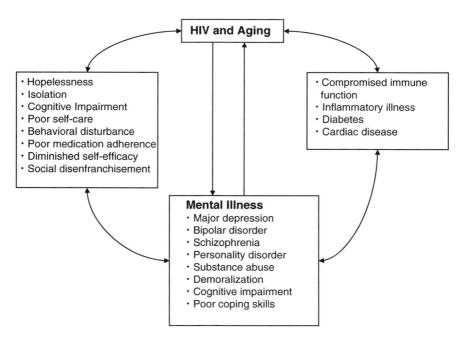

Figure 1 Conceptual framework showing the interrelationship between HIV, aging, mental illness, and medical comorbidities.

showing the relationship between HIV, aging, mental illness, and medical comorbidities that lead to amplification of illness. As a result, older patients with HIV/AIDS have higher morbidity and mortality, with more severe disease at HIV diagnosis, greater risk for HIV-associated complications and illnesses, and shorter survival time (5,6).

Psychiatric disorders occur in elderly populations at increased frequency, including major depression, bipolar affective disorder, dementia, delirium, new-onset schizophrenia, and anxiety disorders. Diagnosis and management of these conditions in older HIV/AIDS patients can be challenging as a result of decreased compliance and adherence to medications.

DEPRESSION

Major depressive disorder (MDD) is the most common psychiatric disorder associated with HIV/AIDS (7). The lifetime prevalence of depression in the general population is estimated at between 5% and 17% as against 22% and 45% in those living with HIV/AIDS (8,9). Whereas the risk of current depression and lifetime depression decreases with age in the general population, there is no difference between old and young individuals with HIV/AIDS (10). A similar trend of lifetime depression rates is observed when comparing homosexual men who were not intravenous drug users (32%), young men with HIV (39%), and older men with HIV (36%) to a significantly lower rate of 20% in HIV-negative older men (11). A meta-analysis showed a twofold increase in risk of depression among HIV-positive samples compared with HIV-negative samples (12). Depression and HIV are interrelated. Depressed individuals are more likely to contract HIV through engaging in risky behavior than nondepressed individuals. These behaviors include having sex for money or drugs, having sex when intoxicated by drugs or alcohol, having sex with intravenous drug users, and having a greater number of sex partners throughout their lifetime (13). Illicit substance abuse is observed to be a stronger risk factor for HIV in psychiatric patients with depressive disorders than in psychiatric patients with other diagnoses (14). HIV-infected persons are more likely to engage in risky behaviors that expose others to HIV (15). Among the elderly, these factors associated with depression translate into increased risk for HIV infection (3). This has implications for HIV/AIDS management in the elderly.

HIV-positive patients with depression surveyed in studies have reported that the onset of depression preceded their knowledge of diagnosis with HIV and, possibly, preceded infection (10). There is evidence to suggest that a new diagnosis of HIV can lead to new-onset depression. In a study of Chinese patients, almost all depressive episodes began after the individuals tested seropositive (16). The stigma of being HIV positive predicts cognitive-affective depression (17) and negative affect in older individuals (18). Worry about HIV is associated with higher depressive symptoms scores (19). Progression of HIV infection is associated with increased likelihood of major depression (20).

Synergistic mechanisms between MDD and HIV may occur because of decreased cobalamin in the brain, thereby increasing the risk of MDD, whose resultant effect is suppression of natural killer (NK) cells and CD8+ T cells, which worsens HIV (21). HIV-positive women with depressive symptoms had lower NK cell activity and higher activated CD8 T lymphocyte levels and viral load (22), and conversely, NK cell activity has been shown to increase when depressive symptoms are reduced (23). HIV-positive females with the lowest CD4 lymphocyte counts and the highest viral load were the most susceptible to depression-related changes (24). Others have postulated that that HIV reduces serotonergic transmission in the brain and thereby increases the risk of depression.

Presently, there is no evidence for distinct subtypes of HIV-related depression other than correlates to personality style, past psychiatric history, and psychosocial circumstances (25). Although the presentation of depression is similar in HIV-positive and HIV-negative individuals, certain symptoms are more common among patients infected with HIV, including sleep and appetite disturbances (26). Decreased energy and libido, on the other hand, are more common among HIV-negative patients (26).

Depression is often underrecognized and underdiagnosed in older patients (27). This is partly because some of the symptoms of depression can also be attributed to normal aging. Underdiagnosis poses more of a problem in the context of HIV infection in the elderly because some symptoms of depression, such as fatigue, decreased appetite and libido, and poor memory, are also symptoms of HIV (2). Distinguishing between these symptoms is important in the elderly, who seek mental health care much less frequently than the younger population (28). HIV-positive adults over the age of 60 years with any mental health care or substance abuse condition, including depression, were less likely to seek behavioral health treatment than their younger counterparts (7).

Depression is associated with disease progression and mortality. A study of HIV-positive women showed that depressed patients were two times more likely to die than individuals without depressive symptoms, even while clinical indicators of disease status were controlled (24). Depressed patients are generally less adherent to their medication regimen than nondepressed patients (29,30). Poor adherence among depressed individuals could be due to self-neglect, apathy, and/or forgetfulness (31). Patients with better adherence to their medication have better virological outcome, greater increase in CD4 lymphocyte count, lower rates of hospitalization (32), and decreased rates of AIDS-related mortality (33).

Depressive symptoms have been identified to be risk factors for poor prognosis through mechanisms other than medical adherence. Depression predicts clinical progression of HIV independently of nonadherence behavior (34). Among patients with poor adherence, mortality rates are higher in those with depressive symptoms than in those without depressive symptoms (35). These adherence-independent effects of depression could result from direct effects of depression on immune system, as well as depression-related behavioral mechanisms.

The elderly continue to have the highest rates of completed suicide among any age group (36), with depression being the most important and treatable risk factor (37). Individuals with HIV and depression may be even more at risk. In a sample of middle-aged and older persons with HIV/AIDS, one in four persons thought about suicide in the week prior to the survey. Individuals who had thoughts of suicide were more likely to have told their close friends about their HIV than those who had no thoughts of suicide (38). Furthermore, people who experience more severe HIV-related symptoms and antiretroviral treatment side effects are more likely to report suicidal ideation (39). Treatment of depression can improve outcome. Women with chronic depressive symptoms who use mental health services have reduced mortality rates (33). HIV-positive patients with depression who are treated with antidepressant medication are more adherent to antiretroviral treatment than those who are not treated with anti-depressants (30). A concerted effort must be made by providers to identify depression or patients with increased risk of depression among the older HIV population and to offer appropriate treatment, thereby reducing the synergestic sequelae of MDD and HIV.

CONCLUSION

HIV/AIDS among the older population proves to be a formidable challenge in the face of mental illness. Unfortunately this population group is endowed with much less resources and social support compared with younger adults living with HIV. There is less awareness and acceptance of HIV in the older population compared with the younger population. Irrespective of age groups, stigma-related experiences have been reported once people learn of an individual's HIV status (40). Time since diagnosis of HIV and current unemployment state are identified to be positively associated with stigma-related experiences. Older adults living with HIV are less likely to be employed and therefore bear the brunt of stigmatization. Older adults may have more fear and negative attitudes toward HIV/AIDS patients resulting from being less knowledgeable about HIV/AIDS, thereby increasing barriers of HIV status disclosure (41). Depression, poor adherence, and HIV status disclosure are associated with stigma-related expe-riences (40). There is a need to bridge the existing gap of HIV intervention programs and services available to older adults when compared with younger adults. A priority must be given to prevention and education in older adults aimed at reducing the rising rates of infections in older adults. Many older adults have long-established sexual practices and may not identify HIV as risk-taking behavior. Surveys in older adult populations revealed that 90% of those who admitted to HIV risk factors did not perceive their risky behavior and therefore had never tested for HIV (42).

Among older adults living with HIV, interventions should be aimed at reducing HIV risk behavior and adherence to medication. Efforts must also be directed toward reducing the negative impact of stigma on HIV-positive older adults, with particular mention of the effects on medication adherence, changes in mood, and disclosure of status to friends and family who can be of support when they learn of a diagnosis of HIV. Cognitive impairment and dementia in older adults with HIV/AIDS pose a challenge with regard to medication adherence and require the employment of medical adherence services. Establishing and expanding present support groups directed toward older adults will provide an environment for patients to feel secure about themselves, increase social support, and provide education about the universal risks of HIV, thereby empowering them to face the challenge of living with HIV. A concerted approach by health care providers is necessary to create an ongoing dialogue with older adults concerning HIV counseling and testing.

HIV/AIDS and mental illness pose a dual threat to our older adult population. Our efforts must be aimed at preventing HIV infections in this age group while at the same time preserving the quality of life of those living with HIV/AIDS. A holistic approach toward health care to mitigate any medical comorbidities and adequate psychiatric treatment are necessary to curb the two-pronged threat in this population. Clinical trials on psychotropic use in older adults with HIV become imperative as the population of HIV patients lives longer and in the face of new infections among older adults.

REFERENCES

1. HIV/AIDS Surveillance Report. Centers for Disease Control and Prevention (CDC) Cases of HIV Infection and AIDS in the United States and Dependent Areas, 2005. Available at: http://www.cdc.gov/hiv/topics/surveillance/resources/reports/2005report/pdf/table8.pdf. Accessed August 18, 2007.
2. el-Sadr W, Gettler J. Unrecognised HIV infection in the elderly. Arch Intern Med 1995; 115(2):184–186.
3. Zablotsky D, Kennedy M. Risk factors and HIV transmission to midlife and older women: knowledge, options, and the initiation of safer sexual practices. J Acquir Immune Defic Syndr 2003; 33(suppl 2):S122–S130.
4. Skapik JT, Treisman GJ. HIV, psychiatric comorbidity, and aging. Clin Geriatrics 2007; 15(3):26–36.
5. Zingmond DS, Kilbourne AM, Justice AC, et al. Differences in symptom expression in the older HIV-positive patients: The Veterans Aging Cohort 3 Site Study and HIV Cost and Service Utilization Study Experience. J Acquir Immune Defic Syndr 2003; 33(suppl 2):S84–S92.
6. Goodkin K, Wilkie FL, Concha M, et al. Aging and neuron-AIDS conditions and changing spectrum of HIV-1 associated morbidity and mortality. J Clin Epidemiol 2001; 54(suppl 1):S35–S43.
7. Zanjani F, Saboe K, Oslin D. Age difference in rates of mental health/substance abuse. AIDS Patient Care STDS 2007; 21(5):347–355.
8. Krishnan KR, Delong M, Kraemer H, et al. Comorbidity of depression with other medical diseases in the elderly. Biol Psychiatry 2002; 52(6):559–588.

9. Kessler RC, Berglund, P, Demler O. Lifetime prevalence and age of onset distributions of DSM-IV disorders in the National Comorbidity Survey Replication. Arch Gen Psychiatry 2005; 62(6):593–602.
10. Justice AC, McGinns KA, Atkinson JH, et al. Psychiatric and neurocognitive disorders among HIV-positive and negative veterans in care: Veterans Aging Cohort Five-Site Study. AIDS 2004; 18(suppl 1):S49–S59.
11. Rabkin JG, McElhiney MC, Ferrando SJ. Mood and substance use disorders in older adults with HIV/AIDS: methodological issues and preliminary evidence. AIDS 2004; 18(suppl 1):S43–S48.
12. Ciesla JA, Roberts JE. Meta-analysis of the relationship between HIV infection and risk for depressive disorders. Am J Psychiatry 2001; 158(5):725–730.
13. Hutton HE, Lyketsos, CG, Zenilman JM, et al. Depression and HIV risk behaviors among patients in a sexually transmitted disease clinic. Am J Psychiatry 2004; 161(5):912–4.
14. Beyer JL, Taylor L, Gersing KR. Prevalence of HIV infection in a general psychiatric outpatient population. Psychosomatics 2007; 48(1):31–37.
15. Angelino AF. Depression and adjustment disorder in patients with HIV disease. Top HIV Med 2002; 10(5):31–35.
16. Jin H, Atkinson JH, Yu X. Depression and suicidality in HIV/AIDS in China. J Affect Disord 2006; 94(1–3):269–275.
17. Simbayi LC, Kalichman S, Strebel A, et al. Internalized stigma, discrimination, and depression among men and women living with HIV/AIDS in Cape Town, South Africa. Soc Sci Med 2007; 64(9):1823–1831.
18. Vance DE. Self-rated emotional health in adults with and without HIV. Psychol Rep 2006; 98(1):106–108.
19. Miles MS, Holditch-Davis D, Pedersen C, et al. Emotional distress in African American women with HIV. J Prev Interv Community 2007; 33(1–2):35–50.
20. Lyketsos CG, Hoover DR, Guccione M, et al. Changes in depressive symptoms as HIV develops. The Multicenter AIDS Cohort Study. Am J Psychiatry 1996; 153:1430–1437.
21. Baldewicz TT, Goodkin K, Blaney NT, et al. Cobalamin level is related to self-reported and clinically rated mood and to syndromal depression in bereaved HIV-1(+) and HIV-1(–) homosexual men. J Psychom Res 2000; 48(2):177–185.
22. Evans DL, Ten Have TR, Douglas, SD, et al. Association of depression with viral load, CD8 T lymphocytes, and natural killer cells in women with HIV infection. Am J Psychiatry 2002; 159(10):1752–1759.
23. Cruess DG, Douglas SD, Petitto JM. Association of resolution of major depression with increased natural killer cell activity among HIV-seropositive women. Am J Psychiatry 2005; 162(11):2125–2130.
24. Ickovics JR, Hamburger ME, Vlahov, D, et al. Mortality, CD4 Cell Count Decline, and Depressive Symptoms among HIV-Seropositive Women. JAMA 2001; 285(11):1466–1474.
25. Judd F, Komiti A, Chua P, et al. Nature of depression in patients with HIV/AIDS. Aust N Z J Psychiatry 2005; 39(9):826–832.
26. Peterkin J, Hintz S, Zisook S. Depression in the context of human immunodeficiency virus infection: implications for treatment. Int Conf AIDS 1990; 6:183.
27. Lebowtiz BD, Pearson JL, Scneider LS, et al. Diagnosis and treatment of depression in late life. Consensus statement update. JAMA 1997; 278(14):1186–1190.

28. Klap R, Unroe KT, Unützer J. Caring for mental illness in the United States: A focus on older adults. Am J Geriatr Psychiatry 2003; 11:517–524.
29. DiMatteo MR, Lepper HS, Croghan TW. Depression is a risk factor for noncompliance with medical treatment. Arch Intern Med 2000; 160(14):2101–2107.
30. Yun LW, Maravi M, Kobayashi JS, et al. Antidepressant treatment improves adherence to antiretroviral therapy among depressed HIV-infected patients. J Acquir Immune Defic Syndr 2005; 38(4):432–438.
31. Singh N, Squier C, Sivek C, et al. Determinants of compliance with antiretroviral therapy in patients with human immunodeficiency virus: prospective assessment with implications for enhancing care. AIDS Care 1996; 8(3):261–269.
32. Paterson DL, Swindells S, Mohr J, et al. Adherence to protease inhibitor therapy and outcomes in patients with HIV infection. Ann Intern Med 2000; 133(1):21–30.
33. Cook JA, Grey D, Burke J, et al. Depressive symptoms and AIDS-related mortality among a multisite cohort of HIV-positive women. Am J Public Health 2004; 94(7): 1133–1140.
34. Bouhnik AD, Préau M, Vincent E, et al. Depression and clinical progression in HIV-infected drug users treated with highly active antiretroviral therapy. Antivir Ther 2005; 10(1):53–61.
35. Lima VD, Geller J, Bangberg DR. The effect of adherence on the association between depressive symptoms and mortality among HIV-infected individuals first initiating HAART. AIDS 2007; 21(9):1175–1183.
36. Arias E, Anderson RN, Kung HC, et al. Deaths: Final Data for 2001. Natl Vital Stat Rep 2003; 52:111–115.
37. Conwell Y, Duberstein PR, Caine ED. Risk factors for suicide in later life. Biol Psychiatry 2002; 52:193–204.
38. Kalichman SC, Heckman T, Kochman A, et al. Depression and thoughts of suicide among middle aged and older persons living with HIV-AIDS. Psychiatr Serv 2000; 51(7):903–907.
39. Carrico AW, Johnson MO, Morin SF, et al. Correlates of suicidal ideation among HIV-positive persons. AIDS 2007; 21(9):1199–1203.
40. Vanable PA, Carey MP, Blair DC, et al. Impact of HIV-related stigma on health behaviors and psychological adjustment among HIV-positive men and women. AIDS Behav. 2006; 10(5):473–482.
41. Schrimshaw EW, Seigel K. Perceived barriers to social support from family and friends among older adults with HIV/AIDS. J Health Psychol 2003; 8(6):738–752.
42. Zelenetz PD, Epstein ME. HIV in the elderly. AIDS Patient Care STDS 1998; 17(4): 255–262.

4

The Cardiovascular System

Kenneth A. Lichtenstein

*Department of Medicine, National Jewish Medical
and Research Center, Denver, Colorado, U.S.A.*

INTRODUCTION

The population infected with HIV, consequent to the use of antiretroviral (ARV) medications, is aging. Questions about cardiovascular disease (CVD) in this population have prompted inquiry (1–4). Cardiovascular events in HIV-positive individuals are uncommon and occur in the background of CVD in the general population. These circumstances have contributed to a number of conflicting findings in this field of study (5–7).

This chapter will initially address CVD in the general population as a point of reference. The similarities and differences regarding the HIV-infected population will be addressed, including HIV pathophysiologic considerations, risk factors, assessment of risk, and management.

CARDIOVASCULAR DISEASE IN THE GENERAL POPULATION

Worldwide, CVD ranks as the most common cause of death, claiming 17.5 million lives per year. This is followed by cancer, respiratory diseases, and HIV/AIDS, each causing 7.6, 4.0, and 2.8 million deaths per year, respectively (8).

PATHOPHYSIOLOGY OF CARDIOVASCULAR DISEASE

General Population

The development of atherosclerotic plaques is multifactorial. Fatty streaks begin forming in the intima media of arteries early in life. This process advances with age. The deposition of atherogenic particles into the intima media of the vessels is related to the size of the particles—smaller lipid particles more easily penetrate the vascular epithelium. Upon deposition into the intima media, these particles transform into immunogenic substances that initiate a cascade of inflammatory cells and production of pro-inflammatory cytokines. Over time the ensuing inflammation then acts to destabilize the fibrous cap of the atheromatous lesion. This can ultimately result in rupture of the endothelium with release of cytokines and prothrombotic substances that can result in obstruction of the vessel lumen with plaque and thrombosis.

The genesis of lipid particles begins in the liver, where very low density lipoprotein (VLDL) is produced. In normal lipid metabolism, VLDL is converted to intermediate-density lipoprotein (IDL), and IDL is further metabolized to low-density lipoprotein cholesterol (LDL-C). Circulating LDL-C is then eliminated by LDL-C receptors. Small amounts of large VLDL (lgVLDL) are also converted to small VLDL (smVLDL). The smaller-sized VLDL and IDL are more easily deposited into the intima media of arteries, along with LDL-C. VLDL, IDL, LDL-C, and triglycerides are often combined in a lipoprotein matrix called apolipoprotein B (ApoB). ApoB is considered the atherogenic component of lipids and can be measured directly in the clinical laboratory.

In atherogenic states greater amounts of smVLDL, IDL, and LDL-C are deposited in the vascular wall. Although triglycerides do not have a significant atherogenic potential, when elevated they can contribute to cardiovascular risk through their association with mechanisms that diminish IDL conversion to LDL-C and that increase smVLDL production, resulting in higher concentrations of ApoB.

The inflammatory component mentioned earlier contributes to the development and destabilization of atherosclerotic plaques. When atherogenic particles infiltrate the artery and are retained in the intima media, they undergo enzymatic and oxidative modifications that result in an inflammatory state. These lipids are then taken up by macrophages that stimulate endothelial cells to express leukocyte adhesion molecules. The macrophages become activated, resulting in the release of pro-inflammatory cytokines such as tumor necrosis factor alpha (TNF-alpha) and interferon gamma, which in turn initiate secretion of interleukin-6 (IL-6) into the circulation while the leukocyte adhesion molecules attract more inflammatory cells to the atherosclerotic plaque (9).

HIV-Infected Population

A number of studies have shown that premature atherosclerosis may be occurring in HIV-infected persons, despite the younger mean age of this group compared with the at-risk general population (1–4). Also, there may be a greater incidence of cardiovascular events in the HIV-infected population of any age group, although this has not been consistently found in all analyses. Studies evaluating surrogate markers of CVD, such as carotid artery intima media thickness and flow-mediated dilation of brachial arteries, have demonstrated a greater amount of atherosclerotic disease in HIV-infected subjects than in age-matched controls (10–12).

Some hypotheses have been proposed to explain the increased risk of CVD in HIV-infected cohorts. The most widely studied hypothesis has assessed the association of specific drugs in each of the ARV classes—nucleoside analogues (NAs), non-nucleoside reverse transcriptase inhibitors (NNRTIs), and protease inhibitors (PIs)—with perturbations of lipids, especially elevations of total cholesterol (TC) and triglycerides (13–17). Some of these agents have also been associated with insulin resistance and visceral fat accumulation (18,19). Paradoxically, other agents (NNRTIs) are associated with elevations of HDL-C (20).

This association, however, does not appear to be solely explained by the toxicity of these drugs. For example, the MACS cohort has been following a large group of subjects at risk for development of HIV infection for over 14 years. Blood specimens were obtained and stored upon entry into the study and then on a periodic basis to the present time. Fifty patients in that cohort became infected with HIV. Lipid panels in those patients were evaluated upon entry into the MACS cohort, at the time of seroconversion, and at six-month intervals thereafter. TC, LDL, and HDL levels all fell below baseline values from the time of HIV seroconversion. When these individuals subsequently initiated highly active ARV therapy (HAART), TC and LDL levels increased to baseline or slightly above baseline levels, and while HDL levels rose, they never returned to their baseline values. When the elevation of levels over the years of follow-up was evaluated, the TC levels appeared to be no different than would have been anticipated had the patients not become HIV infected (21).

Several studies in ARV-naïve patients may support this hypothesis. In all cases, TC, HDL, LDL, and triglyceride levels increased above baseline values, following initiation of ARV. Such findings could suggest a "return to health," an adverse drug effect, or both. A number of additional studies comparing various ARV agents to one another in each class demonstrate relative differences in lipid elevations. In all cases, lipid levels in ARV-naïve patients increase when treatment is initiated; however, both ritonavir and stavudine have been notable for greater elevations in TC and triglycerides than other drugs in their respective classes (22–26).

The difficulty in interpreting these studies is that there is a significant prevalence of dyslipidemias in the general population. The National Health and Nutrition Examination Survey (NHANES) 1999–2000 demonstrated that in the United States, 18% of adults have TC levels greater than 240 mg/dL and 10% of adolescents have TC levels over 200 mg/dL. Forty-eight percent of adult men and 43% of adult women have LDL-C greater than 130 mg/dL. Forty percent of adult men and 15% of adult women have HDL-C less than 40 mg/dL (27). This background prevalence confounds the interpretation of studies in HIV-positive individuals.

There are data suggesting that ARV therapy may be beneficial in the context of CVD. In a subanalysis of a three-arm class-sparing study in ARV-naïve patients utilizing a boosted PI plus two NAs, NNRTIs plus two NAs, and a boosted PI plus an NNRTI, all three regimens resulted in improvements in flow-mediated dilation from the baseline. These results suggest that ARV exerts a beneficial effect on endothelial function (28).

PIs have been implicated as etiologic agents in insulin resistance. To date, few studies have been performed; however, the most consistent finding is that indinavir both induces and sustains a state of insulin resistance (29). Although additional studies have demonstrated some insulin resistance with initiation of other PIs, this condition has not been sustained with continued administration.

The second hypothesis relates to HIV infection. HIV induces a state of chronic inflammation with activation of inflammatory cells and production of pro-inflammatory cytokines independent of the CVD inflammatory process described earlier. The HIV envelope protein, gp120, may activate the smooth muscle tissue factor that may result in endothelial dysfunction, which could further stimulate inflammation. In HIV infection the state of chronic inflammation caused by uncontrolled viral replication may contribute to destabilization of the fibrous cap of the atherosclerotic plaque, leading to rupture and thrombosis (1). Additionally, recent animal studies have shown that Chemokine Co-Receptor 5 (CCR5), the major coreceptor on inflammatory cells for HIV attachment, is also a mediator of the inflammation associated with atherosclerosis (30–33). The nef gene of HIV stimulates the expression of CCR5. These factors, operating together, may make uncontrolled HIV infection an independent risk factor for CVD. Moreover, HIV infection has also been independently associated with the development of insulin resistance, which can lead to the development of diabetes mellitus (34).

CARDIOVASCULAR RISK FACTORS

General Population

The risk of developing a cardiovascular event—acute myocardial infarction (AMI), cerebrovascular accidents (CVA), and peripheral vascular disease (PVD)—is associated with the number of CVD risk factors present in each specific individual. These risk factors include increasing age, hypertension, diabetes mellitus, obesity, dyslipidemia, male sex, smoking, and premature CVD events in first-degree relatives (35,36).

CVD risk increases in a synergistic fashion when two or more of these risk factors are present in an individual. The INTERHEART study demonstrated this by assessing the odds ratios of risk factors associated with AMI in 15,000 AMI patients in comparison with 15,000 control subjects. In this study the risk of experiencing AMI increased in a geometric fashion with the presence of additional risk factors (37).

Some CVD risk factors, such as age, sex, and family history, are not modifiable. Conversely, DM, hypertension, obesity, metabolic syndrome, dyslipidemia, and smoking are all potentially modifiable by incorporation of therapeutic lifestyle changes (TLC) and by treatment of each risk factor with specific pharmacologic agents. Successful modification of these risk factors has been demonstrated in multiple CVD studies to substantially reduce the incidence of cardiovascular events (38–40).

Certain CVD risk factors and combinations of risk factors confer an even greater risk for cardiovascular events. Any three of these five factors—hypertension (≥ 130 mm Hg systolic or ≥ 85 mm Hg diastolic or drug treatment for hypertension), insulin resistance/diabetes mellitus (fasting blood glucose ≥ 100 mg/dL or drug treatment for elevated glucose), elevated triglycerides (≥ 150 mg/dL or drug treatment for elevated triglycerides), reduced HDL-C (<40 mg/dL in men, <50 mg/dL in women, or drug treatment for reduced HDL-C), and elevated waist circumference (≥ 102 cm or 39 inches in men and ≥ 88 cm or 35 inches in women)—constitute the metabolic syndrome. The presence of metabolic syndrome is associated with a disproportionate increase in the risk of AMI (41). Likewise, some risk factors confer a risk for cardiovascular events equivalent to that of having sustained a prior AMI. These are called coronary risk equivalents. Diabetes mellitus, prior CVA, and peripheral artery disease meet this requirement. It is likely that in the near future, grades 3, 4 and 5 renal insufficiency will be included in cardiovascular disease management guidelines as another coronary risk equivalent.

HIV-Infected Population

In the HIV-infected population, the same cardiovascular risk factors are associated with cardiovascular events (1,35,36). However, there are some features that distinguish this group of patients from the general population. In general, this group is younger, has lower rates of hypertension, lower HDL levels, and higher rates of cigarette smoking (37). Two additional factors that may influence cardiovascular risk include HIV infection with its associated chronic inflammation and some of the ARV agents used to treat the infection. In spite of these differences, investigators in the DAD study evaluated their cohort of over 23,000 HIV-infected patients with the Framingham 10-year cardiovascular risk algorithm and found the Framingham model accurately predicted incident myocardial infarction albeit with a slight underestimation that likely reflected the relatively younger age of their cohort (42).

GUIDELINES FOR ASSESSMENT OF CARDIOVASCULAR RISK

Since the risk factors for CVD in HIV-infected individuals are the same as those in the general population, the guidelines for management established by the Infectious Diseases Society of America/AIDS Clinical Group (IDSA/ACTG)

Table 1 National Cholesterol Education Program Adult Treatment Panel III Guidelines for Assessment and Management of Cardiovascular Risk

Risk category	Triglycerides <200 mg/dL			Triglycerides ≥200 mg/dL		
	LDL goal	Lifestyle changes	Drug therapy	Non-HDL-C Goal	Lifestyle changes	Drug therapy
10-year risk >20% or coronary risk equivalent	<100 mg/dL or ≤70 mg/dL	≥100 mg/dL	≥100 mg/dl	<130 mg/dL or ≤100 mg/dL	≥130 mg/dL	≥130 mg/dL
10-year risk 10–20% ≥2 risk factors	<130 mg/dL	≥130 mg/dL	≥130 mg/dL	<160 mg/dL	≥160 mg/dL	≥160 mg/dL
10-year risk <10% ≥2 risk factors	<130 mg/dL	≥130 mg/dL	≥160 mg/dL	<160 mg/dL	≥160 mg/dL	≥160 mg/dL
10-year risk <10% 0–1 risk factor	<160 mg/dL	≥160 mg/dL	≥190 mg/dL	<190 mg/dL	≥190 mg/dL	≥220 mg/dL

are essentially identical to those of the National Cholesterol Education Program Adult Treatment Panel III (NCEP ATP III). The NCEP ATP III guidelines are evidence based and are updated as new information becomes available from large, randomized clinical trials (38–40,43) (Table 1).

TLC remain the backbone of clinical management for all patients. This includes a diet low in saturated fats with increased intake of omega-3 fatty acids, weight control, regular exercise, and avoidance or cessation of cigarette smoking. TLC should be recommended for all patients and emphasized and actively encouraged in those individuals with increased cardiovascular risk.

When two or more CVD risk factors are present, the patients should be evaluated for their 10-year cardiovascular risk. Cardiovascular risk factors incorporated into this assessment include age, sex, presence or treatment of hypertension, diabetes mellitus, obesity, cigarette smoking, and family history of premature cardiovascular events in first-degree relatives (men <55 and women <65 years of age). If two or more of these risk factors are present, the 10-year cardiovascular risk should be calculated using the Framingham or PROCAM algorithm. A 10-year cardiovascular risk score of >20% or the presence of coronary risk equivalents is considered the highest risk. Those individuals with two or more risk factors and a score of 10% to 20% are at moderately high risk, and those with two or more risk factors and a score <10% are considered to be at moderate risk. Those individuals with zero or one risk factor are at lower risk and almost always have a 10-year cardiovascular risk score <10%.

By establishing the 10-year cardiovascular risk, the NCEP ATP III was able to make recommendations for lipid management. In patients with trigly-cerides <200 mg/dL, the LDL-C is the primary target. This is based on large studies that demonstrate a log-linear relationship between the LDL-C level and cardiovascular events. In those individuals with fasting triglycerides >200 mg/dL, non-HDL cholesterol (TC minus HDL) becomes the therapeutic target, and the goal is 30 mg/dL above the LDL-C goal for each risk category. Finally, the tertiary target is HDL-C; however, scientific investigations have not yet been able to establish a specific level above which CVD is reduced (35,36).

High Risk (10-year Risk >20%) or the Presence of Coronary Risk Equivalents

The LDL-C goal in this group is <100 mg/dL. TLC should be initiated if LDL-C is ≥100 mg/dL, and drug therapy should be considered if LDL is ≥100 mg/dL, especially if TLC interventions do not reduce the LDL-C to the goal. For patients with multiple risk factors—especially diabetes mellitus, poorly controlled severe risk factors, and multiple risk factors comprising the metabolic syndrome, acute coronary syndrome, or a baseline LDL of 70 to 100 mg/dL—an LDL-C goal of <70 mg/dL is recommended as an option.

Moderate High Risk (>2 Risk Factors and 10-year Risk 10–20%)

In this group the NCEP ATP III recommends an LDL-C goal of <130 mg/dL with TLC to be initiated if LDL is ≥130 mg/dL, and initiation of lipid-lowering therapy should be considered, especially if the TLC efforts are unsuccessful. The guidelines also suggest that in individuals in this category, whose baseline LDL-C is 100 to 129 mg/dL, an LDL goal of <100 mg/dL is an optional goal.

Moderate Risk (>2 Risk Factors and 10-year Risk <10%)

For these individuals, the guidelines set the LDL-C goal at <130 mg/dL with initiation of TLC at LDL-C ≥130 mg dL. Drug therapy should be considered if LDL-C is ≥160 mg/dL.

Lower Risk (0 or 1 Risk Factor)

Generally, a 10-year cardiovascular risk calculation is rarely necessary because almost all of the individuals in this category have a 10-year risk of <10%. In this group, the LDL-C goal is <160 mg/dL with TLC initiation at LDL-C ≥160 mg/dL. Lipid-lowering therapy is indicated for LDL ≥190 mg/dL and is considered optional for LDL-C levels between 160 and 189 mg/dL.

In all of these cases, it is assumed that the fasting triglyceride level is <200 mg/dL. If the fasting triglyceride level is ≥200 mg/dL, non-HDL cholesterol becomes the goal, and that value is set at 30 mg/dL above the LDL goal in each risk category.

MANAGEMENT OF CARDIOVASCULAR RISK FACTORS

Lipid-lowering therapy is only one facet of CVD prevention. TLC, control of diabetes mellitus, weight reduction, and treatment of hypertension must also be addressed.

TLC include a proper diet, physical activity, weight control, and smoking cessation. Although adherence is difficult, if these interventions are incorporated into the daily routine, they can be effective.

Of seminal importance is the cessation of smoking. This risk factor carries one of the highest risks for CVD. Repetitive vasoconstriction of the segment of the coronary artery adjacent to a hard atherosclerotic plaque physically breaks down the tissues because of the "hinge-like" movement, ultimately resulting in rupture of the vessel at the edge of the plaque. This process also increases the aforementioned inflammatory effects on the atherosclerotic plaque and increases triglyceride levels (9). Permanently removing this risk factor substantially reduces the 10-year cardiovascular risk. Although this is one of the most important risk factors, success rates are low. Furthermore, cohort studies have shown that smoking rates are higher in the HIV-infected population (37,44). A combination of nicotine-replacement drugs or oral agents that reduce the desire to smoke, coupled with formal smoking cessation programs and a decision to cease using cigarettes, has the best success rates.

Exercise and diet together have beneficial effects by reducing the intake of saturated fats, reducing weight, improving insulin resistance, and lowering blood pressure. They have also been shown to have beneficial effects on HDL-C and LDL-C levels (45).

Management of hypertension follows standard guidelines with the use of salt restriction, diuretics, angiotensin-converting enzyme inhibitors (ACEIs), angiotensin receptor blockers (ARBs), and beta blockers. Calcium channel blockers should generally be avoided or, if no alternatives are available, used with caution because they are metabolized via the cytochrome P450 system.

Likewise, treatment of diabetes mellitus and glucose intolerance should be considered vital to maintaining cardiovascular health. As previously mentioned, diabetes mellitus is a coronary risk equivalent. Insulin resistance and type II diabetes mellitus can be managed with diet and insulin-sensitizing agents such as metformin and the glitazones. In type I DM, insulin should be administered in a way that tightly controls blood sugar.

Lipid management should be effected according to NCEP ATP III guidelines. One important caveat regards patients whose triglycerides exceed 400 mg/dL. In these circumstances triglycerides must be brought down below 400 mg/dL with fibrates or omega-3 fatty acids to allow statins to be effective. At these high triglyceride levels, there is an alteration of LDL metabolism, rendering statins much less effective in lowering LDL-C levels. Although it is recommended that caution must be taken when using fibrates and statins together, this is an effective combination—especially when triglycerides have been lowered to <400 mg/dL—but must be monitored closely for adverse events.

Statins are used to bring LDL-C or non-HDL cholesterol to NCEP ATP III goals. In the HIV-infected population, caution must be paramount in their use because most statins are metabolized by the CYP3A4 enzyme system. Since most PIs and delavirdine inhibit that enzyme, statin levels may be elevated to dangerously high levels. Conversely, efavirenz and nevirapine are inducers of the CYP3A4 enzyme system and may lower statin levels to subtherapeutic levels. Lovastatin and simvastatin are contraindicated in individuals taking PIs. Pravastatin has little impact on the CYP3A4 enzyme system, allowing coadministration with PIs. The sole exception is coadministration with darunavir as pravastatin levels can reach toxic levels. Fluvastatin appears to be safe to use with PIs, and atorvastatin and rosuvastatin should be used with caution in patients on PIs by initiating treatment at low doses and gradually titrating upward while monitoring for lipid response and toxicity (46,47).

Ezetemibe can be used to lower LDL-C or non-HDL cholesterol by reducing the absorption of lipids from the gastrointestinal tract. To date, it has been effective in HIV-infected patients and does not appear to interact significantly with ARV agents.

Niacin is useful in raising HDL-C levels. It is best to initiate treatment at lower doses and titrate upward carefully owing to side effects such as flushing. If titrated slowly, these side effects can be minimized or avoided and often subside with continuing use of the drug. Bile acid sequestrants in HIV-infected patients should be avoided since their effect on absorption of ARV agents has not been well characterized and remains a theoretical concern.

ARV Switching

In the HIV-infected population with elevated cardiovascular risk, attention must be paid to ARV agents that can affect lipids. ACTG/IDSA guidelines recommend obtaining a lipid panel prior to initiating ARV therapy (43). If patients are at high risk with ≥2 risk factors or an elevated 10-year cardiovascular risk, then ARV agents known to adversely affect lipids—most often triglycerides—should be avoided. If there are limited choices due to preexisting resistance or intolerance, these ARV agents may be used in conjunction with close lipid monitoring, lipid-lowering drugs, and adherence to NCEP ATP III guidelines. Such an approach could affect medication adherence due to an additional potential for side effects, drug interactions, and the increased burden of multiple medications.

Patients who are already on ARV therapy and have elevated lipids can be managed in one of two ways. In general, TLC and use of lipid-lowering therapy can be undertaken with the precautions previously mentioned. If unsuccessful, ARV therapy can be switched to agents that are more lipid neutral, as long as viral suppression is not compromised. Some specific ARV agents in the NA, NNRTI, or PI class have been associated with lipid abnormalities—specifically elevations of TC and triglycerides. Stavudine can adversely affect lipids. If this is the case, tenofovir or abacavir can replace stavudine if the virus is susceptible to those agents. If ritonavir must be discontinued due to significant elevations in lipid levels—particularly triglycerides—a switch to an NNRTI can be considered, although efavirenz has been associated with lipid elevations in individuals with familial dyslipidemias. Switching to an unboosted PI is generally not recommended, owing to a reduction in effective viral control. As newer agents and classes are developed, they may serve, in part, as effective agents for treatment of HIV infection with less impact on lipids.

SUMMARY

Prevention of CVD in the HIV-infected population should be managed in a fashion similar to that for the general population. CVD risk factors should be evaluated, and if two or more risk factors are present, the 10-year CVD risk should be calculated to obtain the LDL-C goal for patients with triglycerides <200 mg/dL and the non-HDL cholesterol goal for those with triglycerides >200 mg/dL. TLC should be initiated with special attention to smoking cessation, and treatment of modifiable CVD risk factors, such as insulin resistance, diabetes mellitus, hypertension, and obesity, should be initiated. Hyperlipidemia should be managed according to NCEP ATP III guidelines. If triglycerides exceed 400 mg/dL, they must be reduced with fibrates, omega-3 fatty acids, and/or cessation or replacement of drugs that induce elevated triglycerides. In dyslipidemic patients ARV therapy that alters lipids should be avoided. If lipid goals in patients taking these agents cannot be reached with standard interventions or if concerns about adherence to higher pill burdens exist, HIV therapy can be switched to equally effective, lipid-neutral ARV medications.

REFERENCES

1. Currier JS, Taylor A, Boyd F, et al. Coronary heart disease in HIV-infected individuals. JAIDS 2003; 33:506–512.
2. Mary-Krause M, Cotte L, Simon A, et al. Increased risk of myocardial infarction with duration of protease inhibitor therapy in HIV-infected men. AIDS 2003; 17:2479–2486.
3. Passalaris JD, Sepkowitz KA, Glesby MJ. Coronary artery disease and human immunodeficiency virus infection. Clin Infect Dis 2000; 31:787–797.
4. Maggi P, Fiorentino G, Epifani G, et al. Premature vascular lesions in HIV-positive patients: a clockwork bomb that will explode? AIDS 2002; 16:947–948.
5. Friis-Moller N, Sabin R, Weber A, et al. Combination antiretroviral therapy and the risk of myocardial infarction. N Eng J Med 2003; 349:1993–2003.
6. Bozzette SA, Ake CF, Tam HK, et al. Cardiovascular and cerebrovascular events in patients treated for human immunodeficiency virus infection. N Eng J Med 2003; 348: 702–710.

7. El-Sadr WM, Lundgren JD, Neaton F, et al. CD4+ count-guided interruption of antiretroviral treatment. N Eng J Med 2006; 355:2283–2296.
8. World Health Organization. Preventing Chronic Diseases: A Vital Investment 2005. Available at:http:/www.who.int/chp/chronic_disease_report.
9. Hansson GK. Mechanisms of disease: inflammation, atherosclerosis, and coronary artery disease. N Eng J Med 2005; 352(16):1685–1695.
10. Currier JS, Kendall MA, Zackin R, et al. Carotid artery intima-media thickness and HIV infection: traditional risk factors overshadow impact of protease inhibitor exposure. AIDS 2005; 19:927–933.
11. Solages A, Vita JA, Thornton DJ, et al. Endothelial function in HIV-infected persons. Clin Infect Dis 2006; 42:1325–1332.
12. Hsue PY, Lo JC, Franklin A, et al. Progression of atherosclerosis as assessed by carotid intima-media thickness in patients with HIV infection. Circulation 2004; 109:1603–1608.
13. Martinez E, Domingo P, Galindo MJ, et al. Risk of metabolic abnormalities in patients infected with HIV receiving antiretroviral therapy that contains lopinavir-ritonavir. Clin Infect Dis 2004; 38:1017–1023.
14. Friis-Moller N, Reiss P, Sabin CA, et al. Class of antiretroviral drugs and the risk of myocardial infarction. N Eng J Med 2007; 356:1723–1735.
15. Holmberg SD, Moorman AC, Williamson JM, et al. Protease inhibitors and cardiovascular outcomes in patients with HIV-1. Lancet 2002; 360:1747–1748.
16. Gutierrez F, Padilla S, Navarro A, et al. Lopinavir plasma concentrations and changes in lipid levels during salvage therapy with lopinavir/ritonavir-containing regimens. JAIDS 2003; 33:594–600.
17. Grubb JR, Dejam A, Voell J, et al. Lopinavir-Ritonavir: effects on endothelial cell function in healthy subjects. J Infect Dis 2006; 193:1516–1519.
18. Vigouroux C, Gharakhanian S, Sahli Y, et al. Adverse metabolic disorders during highly active antiretroviral treatment (HAART) of HIV disease. Diabetes Metab 1999; 24:383–392.
19. Carr A, Samaras K, Burton S, et al. A syndrome of peripheral lipodystrophy, hyperlipidaemia, and insulin resistance in patients receiving HIV protease inhibitors. AIDS 1998; 12:F51–F58.
20. Negredo E, Ribalta J, Ferre R, et al. Efavirenz induces a striking and generalized increase of HDL-cholesterol in HIV-infected patients. AIDS 2004; 18:819–821.
21. Riddler SA, Smit E, Cole SR, et al. Impact of HIV infection and HAART on serum lipids in men. JAMA 2003; 289(22):2978–2982.
22. Eron J, Yeni P, Gathe J, et al. The KLEAN study of fosamprenavir-ritonavir versus lopinavir-ritonavir, each in combination with abacavir-lamivudine, for initial treatment of HIV infection over 48 weeks: a randomized non-inferiority trial. Lancet 2006; 368:476–482.
23. Johnson M, Grinsztejn B, Rodriguez C, et al. Atazanavir plus ritonavir or saquinavir, and lopinavir/ritonavir in patients experiencing multiple virological failures. AIDS 2005; 19:685–694.
24. van Leth F, Phanuphak P, Stroes E, et al. Nevirapine and efavirenz elicit different changes in lipid profiles in antiretroviral-therapy-naive patients infected with HIV-1. PloS Med 2004; 1:64–74.
25. Gallant J, DeJesus D, Arribas JR, et al. Tenofovir DF, Emtricitabine, and Efavirenz vs. Zidovudine, Lamivudine, and Efavirenz for HIV. N Eng J Med 2006; 354:251–260.

26. Montes ML, Pulido F, Barros C, et al. Lipid disorders in antiretroviral-naive patients treated with lopinavir/ritonavir-based HAART: frequency, characterization and risk factors. J Antimicrob. Chemotherapy 2005; 55:800–804.
27. Ford ES, Mokdad AH, Giles WH, et al. Serum total cholesterol concentrations and awareness, treatment, and control of hypercholesterolemia among U.S. adults. Findings from the National Health and Nutrition Examination Survey, 1999–2000. Circulation 2003; 107(17):2185–2189.
28. Torriani FJ, Parker FA, Murphy FL, et al. Antiretroviral therapy improves endothelial function in treatment-naïve HIV-infected subjects. 10th EACS, 2005; Dublin (abstract P55.3).
29. Noor MA, Seneviratne FT, Aweeka JC, et al. Indinavir acutely inhibits insulin-stimulated glucose disposal in humans: a randomized, placebo-controlled study. AIDS 2002; 16:F1–F8.
30. Potteaux S, Combadiere C, Esposito B, et al. Role of bone marrow-derived CC-chemokine receptor 5 in the development of atherosclerosis of low-density lipoprotein receptor knockout mice. Arterioscler Thromb Vasc Biol 2006; 23(8):1858–1863.
31. Bursill CA, Channon KM, Greaves DR. The role of chemokines in atherosclerosis: recent evidence from experimental models and population genetics. Curr Opin Lipidol 2004; 15(2):145–149.
32. Tacke F, Alvarez D, Kaplan TJ, et al. Monocyte subsets differentially employ CCR2, CCR5, and CX3CR1 to accumulate within atherosclerotic plaques. J Clin Invest 2007; 117(1):89–93.
33. Dyfeld J, Bogdanski P, Pupek-Musialik D, et al. Expression of chemokine receptor CCR5 in patients with type 2 diabetes. Pol Merkur Lekarski 2006; 20(116):195–198.
34. El-Sadr WM, Mullin CM, Carr A, et al. Effects of HIV disease on lipid, glucose and insulin levels: results from a large antiretroviral-naïve cohort. HIV Med 2005; 6: 114–121.
35. Grundy SM, Cleeman JI, Merz C, et al. Implications of recent clinical trials for the National Cholesterol Education Program Adult Treatment Panel III Guidelines. Circulation 2004; 110:227–239.
36. Anonymous. Third Report of the National Cholesterol Education Program (NCEP) Expert Panel on Detection, Evaluation, and Treatment of High Blood Cholesterol in Adults (Adult Treatment Panel III): final report. Circulation 2002; 106:3143–3421.
37. Yusuf S, Hawken S, Ounpuu S, et al. Effect of potentially modifiable risk factors associated with myocardial infarction in 52 countries (the INTERHEART study): case-control study. Lancet 2004; 364:937–952.
38. Heart Protection Study Collaborative Group. MRC/BHF Heart Protection Study of cholesterol lowering with simvastatin in 20536 high-risk individuals: a randomized placebo-controlled trial. Lancet 2002; 360(9326):7–22.
39. ALLHAT Officers and Coordinators for the ALLHAT Collaborative Research Group. The Antihypertensive and Lipid-Lowering Treatment to Prevent Heart Attack Trial. Major outcomes in moderately hypercholesterolemic, hypertensive patients randomized to pravastatin vs. usual care: The Antihypertensive and Lipid-Lowering Treatment to Prevent Heart Attack Trial (ALLHAT-LLT). JAMA 2002; 288: 2998–3007.

40. Severs PS, Dahlof B, Poulter NR, et al. Prevention of coronary and stroke events with atorvastatin in hypertensive patients who have average or lower-than average cholesterol concentrations, in the Anglo-Scandinavian Cardiac Outcomes Trial-Lipid Lowering Arm (ASCOT-LLA): a multicentre randomized controlled trial. Lancet 2003; 361:1149–1158.

41. Grundy SM, Cleeman JI, Daniels SR, et al. Diagnosis and management of the metabolic syndrome. An American Heart Association/National Heart, Lung, and Blood Institute Scientific Statement. Executive Summary. Circulation. 2005; 112:1–6.

42. Law MG, Griis-Moller N, El-Sadr WM, et al. The use of the Framingham equation to predict myocardial infarctions in HIV-infected patients: comparison with observed events in the D:A:D Study. HIV Med 2006; 7(4):218.

43. Dube MP, Stein JH, Aberg JA, et al. Guidelines for the evaluation and management of dyslipidemia in HIV-infected adults receiving antiretroviral therapy. Recommendations of the HIV Medical Association of the Infectious Disease Society of America and the Adult AIDS Clinical Trials Group. Clin Infect Dis. 2003; 37:613–627.

44. Saves M, Chene G, Ducimetiere P, et al. Risk factors for coronary heart disease in patients treated for human immunodeficiency virus infection compared with the general population. Clin Infect Dis 2003; 37:292–298.

45. Stafenick ML, Mackey MS, Sheehan M, et al. Effects of diet and exercise in men and postmenopausal women with low levels of HDL cholesterol and high levels of LDL cholesterol. NEJM 1998; 339(1):12–20.

46. Shepherd J, Blauw GJ, Murphy MB, et al. Pravastatin in elderly individuals at risk of vascular disease (PROSPER): a randomized controlled trial. PROspective Study of Pravastatin in the Elderly at Risk. Lancet 2002; 360:1623–1630.

47. Cannon CP, Braunwald E, McCabe CH, et al. Intensive versus moderate lipid lowering with statins after acute coronary syndromes. N Eng J Med 2004; 350:1495–1504.

5

The Endocrine System

Ruth M. Greenblatt

*Departments of Clinical Pharmacy, Medicine, Epidemiology
and Biostatistics, University of California, San Francisco, California, U.S.A.*

Phyllis C. Tien

*Department of Medicine, University of California, and Department
of Veterans Affairs, San Francisco, California, U.S.A.*

INTRODUCTION

Effective antiretroviral therapy has improved survival after detection of HIV infection from 4 to 24 years (1). It is anticipated that HIV infection will increasingly coexist with conditions associated with aging. Several metabolic and endocrine disorders that are closely associated with aging are also associated with HIV infection, and there is a potential for adverse synergy between aging and metabolic diseases. To further complicate matters, several antiretroviral medications may also perturb metabolism, so the potential interactions between aging, HIV infection, and its treatment are producing a complex and rapidly evolving clinical knowledge base. Increasingly, HIV care providers will need to diagnose and treat endocrine and metabolic diseases of aging, including loss of peripheral subcutaneous fat and increases in axial fat, type 2 diabetes mellitus (DM) and insulin resistance, hypogonadism, hypothyroidism, osteoporosis, and osteonecrosis.

FAT DISTRIBUTION CHANGES

Fat distribution changes were first reported in HIV-infected individuals soon after the advent of effective antiretroviral therapy (2–6). The changes that were most commonly observed included fat accumulation (or lipohypertrophy) in central sites, including the abdomen and upper back, and in women, breast, and fat loss (or lipoatrophy) in peripheral sites, particularly in the leg, arm, buttock, and face; fat changes were often accompanied by insulin resistance and dyslipidemia. These changes in HIV infection were described as a "lipodystrophy syndrome" in 1998 (2). The protease inhibitor (PI) class of antiretroviral drugs was most often implicated, because the introduction of these drugs appeared to coincide with the appearance of fat and metabolic changes. A sex difference was also suggested in early reports (7–10), with central lipohypertrophy being more common in HIV-infected women.

More recent studies have found that peripheral lipoatrophy appears to be the predominant syndrome associated with HIV infection in both men and women (11–14). Studies in HIV-infected men (11) and women (12), using MRI-measured regional adipose tissue, show that HIV infection appears to be associated with subcutaneous fat loss that is particularly marked in the lower trunk and leg when compared with mainly HIV-uninfected controls. These studies also found that there was no reciprocal increase in visceral fat, as had been suggested in early reports (11,12).

Contrary to early reports, a prospective study in HIV-infected women found that the risk of central lipohypertrophy over a two-and-a-half-year period was similar to that in HIV-uninfected women, suggesting that the observed increase may be a result of normal aging (14). Similar findings were also observed in a prospective study of HIV-infected men, where increases in waist circumference were similar in HIV-infected and uninfected men, while the increase in hip circumference in HIV-infected men over time was less than in uninfected men (15). Another study in antiretroviral-naïve HIV-infected men who were started on highly active antiretroviral therapy demonstrated increases in leg fat and trunk fat as measured by dual X-ray absorptiometry (DXA) scans during the first 24 weeks on therapy, suggesting a restoration to health phenomenon (16). In the subsequent weeks, decreases in leg fat were observed while trunk fat remained stable.

These recent studies conflict with early reports likely because most early reports defined body fat changes using a dichotomous outcome of presence or absence of lipodystrophy, rather than a continuous measure of regional fat (17). Lipodystrophy was defined using subjective criteria of participant report of fat change with or without confirmation by clinical exam. Most early studies also did not include a comparison group of uninfected patients. Data comparing HIV-infected men and women must also be interpreted with caution in the absence of respective uninfected comparison groups, since women in general have more body fat than men.

Accumulating evidence also shows that the nucleoside reverse transcriptase inhibitor (NRTI) class and, in particular, the drug stavudine is most associated with lipoatrophy (11,12,16,18). The association with stavudine has been further supported by studies, which have shown that the discontinuation of stavudine or substitution of stavudine with another NRTI has led to partial improvements in leg fat loss, although not to baseline levels (19–23). A study in HIV-infected women found that discontinuation of stavudine led to slower decreases in the mean annual change in thigh and hip circumference compared with those who stayed on stavudine; HIV-uninfected women, on the other hand, continued to demonstrate increases. The findings of these studies suggest that there is likely a direct effect of HIV infection itself on lipoatrophy. On the other hand, the substitution of a PI with a non-nucleoside reverse transcriptase inhibitor (NNRTI) or abacavir has not led to improvements in fat (24,25).

The biologic mechanism most often studied to explain the association of stavudine with lipoatrophy is mitochondrial toxicity. Stavudine is thought to inhibit mitochondrial DNA polymerase gamma, the enzyme necessary for the replication of mitochondrial DNA (26). Using electron microscopy, mitochondrial damage has been found within subcutaneous fat, as well as decreased levels of mitochondrial DNA and mitochondrial-encoded proteins (27). Mitochondrial DNA depletion also appears more pronounced in stavudine-treated patients (28).

Other than discontinuation of stavudine, there are currently few, if any, effective therapies to reverse lipoatrophy. Several clinical trials have studied the use of thiazolidinediones, such as rosiglitazone, but the data have been conflicting (29–32). Another small study found that the HMG-coA reductase inhibitor pravastatin given for 12 weeks was associated with increases in both limb and abdominal subcutaneous fat (33). The authors hypothesized that lipoatrophy might be the result of an inflammatory process, which might be reversed with a statin. Uridine supplementation has also been studied in a small pilot study and shown to improve lipoatrophy (defined by patient report confirmed by clinical exam) (34). The rationale for studying uridine is that the drug might attenuate the mitochondrial DNA decline by preventing apoptosis secondary to pyrimidine decline. Finally, interval injections of polylactic acid, a biosynthetic polymer, have been used for facial lipoatrophy in HIV-infected individuals and have led to increases in quality of life (35,36).

Older age has been independently associated with lipoatrophy in several HIV studies (11,12,37–39). In one cross-sectional study of HIV-infected men (11) and women (12) that used direct measures of regional adipose tissue, older age was associated with less subcutaneous fat in the leg in HIV-infected men and a trend toward a decrease in HIV-infected women. In these studies, older age was also associated with more visceral adipose tissue (VAT) in HIV-infected men and women. Central obesity and, to a lesser extent, decreases in peripheral fat have been reported in the normal population with aging. Whether or not aging will exacerbate HIV-associated peripheral fat loss is unclear.

DISORDERS OF GLUCOSE METABOLISM

Disorders in glucose metabolism, including insulin resistance and DM, have been of increased concern since the introduction of antiretroviral therapy. Prior to the highly active antiretroviral therapy (HAART) era, a study comparing insulin sensitivity in HIV-infected patients with healthy controls with similar body composition found that HIV infection was associated with increased insulin sensitivity (40). Another study found no difference in insulin sensitivity between antiretroviral-naïve HIV-infected and control patients (41). A 3.3% prevalence of self-reported DM was also demonstrated in a study of antiretroviral-naïve HIV-infected patients with a mean age of 38 years compared with 5.9% reported by the United States Public Health Service for patients of similar age (42). These studies suggest that HIV infection per se is not associated with disorders in glucose metabolism.

Among the antiretroviral drugs, several studies have found an association between PI use and insulin resistance in HIV-infected individuals (2,41,43,44). One study, by showing that changes in glucose and insulin occurred before the onset of fat changes, demonstrated that the effect of PI on insulin resistance was independent of fat changes (45). In vitro studies have also demonstrated a direct inhibitory effect of certain PIs on cellular glucose transport (46). In HIV-uninfected volunteers, acute decreases in insulin sensitivity were also observed after a single dose of the PI, indinavir (47), or lopinavir/ritonavir (48).

However, the acute decrease in insulin sensitivity observed after a single dose of PI in studies of HIV-infected volunteers may be transient. PI use for more than four weeks appeared to ameliorate the observed acute induction of insulin resistance. In one study, the acute decrease in insulin sensitivity observed after a single dose of lopinavir/ritonavir was not apparent after four weeks on lopinavir/ritonavir (49). In another study, the acute decrease in insulin sensitivity observed after a single dose of indinavir (47) appeared reduced in those given indinavir for four weeks (50). A possible explanation for the improvement in insulin sensitivity in these studies was the observed increases in levels of the adipocyte hormone adiponectin from the baseline after four weeks of therapy. Adiponectin is associated with increased insulin sensitivity.

Large prospective studies have found that regardless of which HAART regimen (PI-containing, NNRTI-containing, or PI- plus NNRTI-containing) an antiretroviral-naïve patient began, insulin levels increased over a median of five years (51). Other prospective studies have demonstrated an association of longer cumulative use of NRTI with insulin resistance in HIV-infected men (52) and DM in HIV-infected women (53). The NRTIs stavudine and lamivudine have been most often implicated (52,53).

Older age has also been associated with DM (51–53) and decreased insulin sensitivity (54) in HIV-infected individuals. Two cross-sectional studies—one in middle-aged HIV-infected women (54) and the other in older HIV-infected men older than 49 years (55)—found a substantial prevalence of self-reported

DM of 13% and 18%, respectively. The increased prevalence could be attributed to patients in these studies being on HAART. Although, on multivariable analysis of the HIV-infected women, HAART was no longer associated with DM, traditional risk factors such as obesity, family history of DM, and decreased physical activity were associated (54). Both increased body mass index and decreased physical activity are common with aging.

Abdominal obesity is recognized to be associated with disorders in glucose metabolism in the aging population and has also been associated with HIV-infected individuals. A cross-sectional study in HIV-infected individuals demonstrated an association between visceral fat and upper trunk subcutaneous adipose tissue with insulin resistance, which was also similarly demonstrated in a comparison group of mainly HIV-uninfected controls (56). Interestingly, in addition to visceral fat, subcutaneous fat in the upper trunk may also be metabolically active. Other studies have also shown an association between waist circumference and insulin resistance, impaired glucose tolerance, and diabetes in HIV-infected individuals (54,57).

The alterations in body fat changes that are observed with aging may be partly mediated through changes in sex hormone levels. In HIV-uninfected postmenopausal women, estrogen supplementation has been associated with maintenance of gynoid fat distribution (or increased lower trunk, hip, thigh, and leg fat), as opposed to android fat distribution (or increased upper trunk and neck fat and decreased hip, thigh, and leg fat) in those not receiving estrogen supplementation (58). Some studies suggest that HIV-infected women may undergo the transition to menopause earlier in age than normal healthy women, which could potentially accelerate the body fat changes associated with HIV infection and increase the risk for glucose abnormalities. In postmenopausal women, testosterone levels have also been shown to rise.

In men, aging is associated with decreases in testosterone levels that have in turn been associated with increases in abdominal obesity (59). In HIV infection, low testosterone levels have been observed in HIV-infected men and women. Low testosterone levels more pronounced in those with the "wasting syndrome" (which generally refers to muscle wasting as opposed to fat wasting) (60).

Endogenous hormones, particularly testosterone, have been associated with DM in the HIV-uninfected population, and there appears to be a sex dimorphism in this association (61). In women, high testosterone levels in premenopausal (mainly from hyperandrogenic conditions, as seen in polycystic ovarian syndrome) and postmenopausal women have been associated with glucose intolerance and insulin resistance. Testosterone levels are thought to increase on menopause due to the loss of estrogen inhibition. On the other hand, in men, low testosterone appears to be associated with insulin resistance (59,62). While it has been hypothesized that testosterone levels might influence insulin sensitivity through their effects on body fat, some studies in men (62) and women (61) have found an independent effect of endogenous hormones. Little is known about the association of testosterone levels and disorders of glucose metabolism in HIV-infected men, but data from the normal population suggest that the hypogonadism observed in some HIV-infected men may be associated with an increased risk for metabolic complications.

MENOPAUSE AND "ANDROPAUSE"

Gonadal Aging in Men

Androgen levels, especially free or unbound androgen levels, decline steadily with age, beginning in early adulthood. The typical changes of aging in men—decreases in strength, fitness, libido, cognitive function, lean body (muscle) mass, and bone density and increases in total body and abdominal fat—also occur among younger men who have low serum testosterone levels (<250–300 ng/mL). The existence and importance of a syndrome of partial androgen deficiency of aging men (PADAM) is controversial. It is not clear whether diminished androgen levels cause these changes, although testosterone replacement in younger men with low serum levels results in increased muscle mass and strength and some improvement in cognitive function (63).

Studies of testosterone replacement in older men have given mixed results, providing little clear evidence for treatment recommendations. Besides mixed evidence of the efficacy of androgen treatment in PADAM, the potential risks of these treatments merit careful consideration. Evaluation and treatment of male hypogonadism with aging in the setting of HIV infection is confounded by lack of clear evidence–based direction.

Studies of PADAM in general and studies of androgen deficiency in HIV and treated HIV infection have yielded conflicting findings. Greater CD4 T-cell depletion, body weight, and age were associated with lower free testosterone levels in pre-HAART HIV-infected men, but low free testosterone levels in one clinical trial study was uncommon among middle-aged HIV-infected men prior to initiation of HAART, and levels tend to increase once HAART is initiated (64). In contrast, another study found low free testosterone levels in 44% of adults prior to HAART and no improvement in the levels on HAART (65). Neither study specified that specimens were obtained in the morning, nor were multiple specimens pooled to eliminate the effects of pulsatility, so some of these differences might be explained by diurnal variation or method of specimen sampling. Recreational drug use may underlie some of the conflicting study results. It has been shown that use of cocaine and opiates is associated with low free testosterone levels in both men and women (66).

Studies have shown low free testosterone levels, often with normal or low luteinizing hormone levels (indicating secondary hypogonadism) among HIV-infected men, which may not improve after successful HAART (65,67). Erectile dysfunction is also common and more prevalent among men with low CD4 cell counts, depression, and advancing age (68) but not necessarily in association with hypogonadism. Klein and colleagues studied 502 HIV-infected and HIV-uninfected men over age 49 and found that hypogonadism, defined by total testosterone levels less than 300 ng/dL, was present in half and independently associated with recent injection drug use, hepatitis C coinfection, indicators of HIV morbidity, and receipt of psychotropic medications. Whether in young HIV-infected men with wasting or older hypogonadal men, the administration of testosterone is associated with increases in total and lean body mass (69); however, megestrol acetate is at least as effective (64). Changes in lean body mass and decreases in subcutaneous fat have been reported by multiple studies of exogenous testosterone, but visceral fat mass does not improve (70). Anemia was associated with low total testosterone levels in one study of HIV-infected men who had fairly low CD4 T-cell nadir values, while those on treatment with antiretroviral therapy (ART) or supplemental androgens had less anemia (71).

Diagnosis

On physical examination, male hypogonadism may be characterized by testicular atrophy, changes in hair growth, and gynecomastia. Peak testosterone levels occur in the morning. Testing with a mixture of three blood samples, each collected 10 minutes apart during the morning, has been advocated because secretion is pulsatile. The most common assay is total serum testosterone, including protein-bound hormone, which may be proportionately increased in HIV infection. Measurement of free testosterone has been advocated when total testosterone levels are low to normal. Depending on setting and level of suspicion, evaluation of pituitary/hypothalamic function may be indicated, though for most HIV patients, etiology of hypogonadism is not identifiable. Among patients with low CD4 cell counts, opportunistic infection and AIDS malignancies should be considered in the differential diagnoses of primary (testicular) and secondary (pituitary/hypothalamic) male hypogonadism.

While the possibly rejuvenating properties of androgen treatments have been advocated, these treatments may have significant risks, particularly in the setting of HIV infection. Recognized adverse effects of androgens include increased risk of prostate cancer, possible increase in thrombotic events and cardiovascular disease, hepatotoxicity (especially with orally administered formulations), priapism, gynecomastia, sleep apnea, and acne. Endogenous androgens also cause thymic involution (72). Androgen deprivation therapy, used for prostate cancer, shows enhanced thymic regeneration with thymopoiesis and improved function of other components of the immune system. In the setting of prostate cancer, androgen blockade and renewed thymopoiesis may have the benefit of invigoration of host responses to abnormal cells (72).

In the setting of HIV infection, exogenous androgens may reduce ongoing thymopoiesis, which may be particularly important to immune reconstitution after initiation of HAART. Use of exogenous androgens, thus, could impede immunologic recovery in HIV infection, though information on this important topic is very limited.

Gonadal Aging in Women

While hypogonadism does not occur uniformly among men, cessation of ovarian function occurs in all women at an average age of 52 years. Few studies have provided information on the effects of menopause on the course of HIV infection. The influence of menopause on immune responses in HIV is biologically plausible since sex and age influence immune responses, and these can be clinically significant as evidenced in autoimmune diseases and some infections (73–82). Sex steroids influence both adaptive and innate immune functions (83–85), but as Cu-Uvin noted in 2005, there is a paucity of data on hormonal levels in HIV-infected women (86). In women, the ovulatory cycle and menopause are major determinants of sex steroid levels. Sex and the female sex steroids estrogen and progesterone have broad effects on lymphocyte numbers, proportions, and functions (87–91). Premenopausal females tend to have stronger T-cell responses than males, though dimorphisms of both response and adverse event rates have been reported in both directions (80,92). A combined analysis from the European and Swiss Cohorts reported lower CD4 cell counts among women who reported menopause, though rate of CD4 decline did not differ by menopausal status (93). Clark et al. reported that CD4 cell counts were somewhat lower among women who lacked evidence of recent ovulation (94) after an analysis of the participants of several ACTG protocols.

Most of the published studies on menopause among HIV-infected women have focused on the effects of HIV on menopause and menopausal symptoms (95–97). Menopause is most often defined by the existing "gold standard": the last menstrual period occurring more than 12 months previously. This definition has its limits: it is based on self-report, and it is subject to misclassification because it makes no distinction between prolonged amenorrhea (with a variety of causes) and menopause (due to depletion of ovarian follicles). Since amenorrhea is common in illness, HIV would be expected to be associated with the cessation or interruption of menses, and it is (98). Women in late middle age who experience amenorrhea from any cause are more likely than younger women to report menopause. Therefore, in the setting of chronic illness, self-reported menopause may not be accurate. The WIHS study group has found self-reported menopause can be transient (it resolves when menses recur) and is not consistently associated with biologic indicators of ovarian function. Several published studies of the effects of HIV on menopausal symptoms have found associations between HIV infection and symptoms that are attributed to menopause, such as depression, arthralgia, and sweats, which were also associated with more profound CD4 T-cell depletion (96,99). Because these symptoms are not specific for menopause and could also be associated with HIV disease progression, current findings do not clearly indicate that HIV influences age at menopause or menopausal symptoms. Studies that demonstrate an association between HIV infection and menopause also show that CD4 cell count depletion was the strongest predictor, indicating that amenorrhea of chronic illness may be the underlying process.

There is no reason to expect hormone replacement therapy to have special benefits or indications in the setting of HIV infection. Hypothetically, exogenous sex steroid treatments could contribute to thymic involution and thus impair production of naïve lymphocytes and the vigor of immune responses, though studies on this have not been done. Androgen supplementation in premenopausal HIV-infected women with low pretreatment testosterone levels and weight loss did not produce adverse effects on glucose tolerance but only had modest effects on lean and fatty tissues (100).

THYROID FUNCTION

Regulation of thyroid hormone production is influenced by aging, chronic illness, inflammatory illness, and autoimmunity to thyroid tissues, all of which are considerations in the setting of HIV infection. While only a small number of studies have examined the impact of HIV infection on thyroid function, in general there is relatively little indication of major effects (101). Since wasting and chronic illness can be associated with HIV infection, the "euthyroid sick syndrome," in which both thyroid stimulating hormone (TSH) and thyroxine (T4) levels are reduced, can be associated with HIV disease, usually advanced illness. Thyroiditis due to opportunistic pathogens in HIV has been identified via thyroid tissue aspirates in the setting of primary hypothyroidism, usually accompanied by localizing symptoms in the neck and other systemic signs of infection (102–106).

Autoimmune phenomena have been long recognized in HIV infection. Mulitple pathogenic mechanisms have been implicated in autoimmune thyroid diseases, including the presence of antithyroid antibody with TSH receptor agonist activity and tissue injury related to thyroid-specific, and nonspecific, CD4 and CD8 cell activation. While apparently uncommon, delayed Grave's syndrome–like presentations have been reported one to three years after HAART initiation characterized by decreased TSH and increased free T4 and triiodothyronine (T3) levels. The development of antithyroid antibodies has been observed in some of these cases. Post-HAART, Grave's disease appears to differ from other "immune reconstitution" phenomena that follow HAART initiation, in that the thyroid abnormalities occur later in time (a year or more after treatment initiation) (107). Similar phenomena have been reported among recipients of IL-2 treatment for HIV, supporting the concept that immunologic factors may cause Grave's syndrome in the setting of HAART immune reconstitution (102). While multiple case series of post-HAART development of antithyroid antibodies have been published (107–110), the incidence of autoimmune thyroiditis after HAART appears to be low (111). One case series found hyperthyroidism to be more common than hypothyroidism among a group of ethnically Chinese patients with good virologic responses to HAART. In this group, antimicrosomal antibodies were more common than antithyroid antibodies (112). Overall, subclinical hypothyroidism appears to be the most common form of thyroid disease in HIV patients, including HAART recipients (111,113,114).

In the absence of signs and symptoms of hyper- or hypothyroidism and clinical findings of a focal process such as thyroiditis or nodules, HIV patients should be screened for thyroid dysfunction as recommended for healthy adults; beginning at 35 years of age, measurement of serum TSH should occur every 5 years (115). While thyroid disease is 10 times more common among women than men, the American Thyroid Association recommends screening in both sexes (115). Clinicians should be particularly alert for clinical hyperthyroidism and Grave's disease during the first years of HAART therapy, since an immune reconstitution syndrome, while rare, may be more common during this time period.

DISORDERS IN BONE METABOLISM

Osteoporosis and osteopenia have been increasingly recognized in HIV-infected individuals since the advent of effective antiretroviral therapy and, like other fat and metabolic changes, were attributed early on to protease inhibitors. In the general population, osteoporosis and osteopenia are important predictors of fragility fractures. A recent meta-analysis of published cross-sectional studies found that the prevalence of osteoporosis was about 15% in HIV-infected individuals—three times the prevalence in HIV-uninfected individuals (116).

Osteoporosis and osteopenia have generally been defined using the World Health Organization criteria, which categorize bone mineral density (BMD) measured on dual X-ray energy absorptiometry (DXA) scanning into two groups. Osteoporosis is defined as a T score less than –2.5 and indicates that the BMD is less than 2.5 standard deviations of the mean BMD of a young healthy population adjusted for sex and race. Osteopenia is defined as a T score between –2.5 and –1 standard deviation. These criteria were established to compare BMD in postmenopausal women to a young healthy population, but have been commonly used in studies of HIV-infected individuals.

Early studies in HIV-infected individuals suggested that PIs may be associated with reduced BMD (117–119). Subsequent studies found that HIV-infected patients on antiretroviral therapy (regardless of type) had reduced BMD when compared with antiretroviral-naïve patients (117,120–122). In longitudinal studies that included ART-experienced HIV-infected patients, reduced BMD was highly prevalent, but over time the BMD either increased or remained stable, after controlling for other factors associated with reduced BMD (118,123–125). In longitudinal studies that included ART-naïve HIV-infected patients, BMD appeared to decrease (16,126). In one of these studies, ART-naïve HIV-infected patients were randomized to a stavudine, lamivudine, and efavirenz or a tenofovir, lamivudine, and efavirenz arm. Those in the tenofovir arm had greater decreases in BMD than in those in the stavudine arm (–2.2% vs. –1.0%, respectively; $P < 0.001$), suggesting that specific ART drugs might be associated with reduced BMD (126).

Several studies have also compared HIV-infected patients to uninfected patients and found that HIV infection is associated with reduced BMD (117, 119–121,127–129). The proposed mechanism by which HIV infection per se may lead to reduced BMD includes cytokine activation due to chronic HIV infection leading to increased bone resorption (130). Increases in tumor necrosis factor (TNF) may partly explain the effect of HIV infection on bone resorption, because of the association between TNF and advanced HIV (131) and because markers of bone resorption appear to correlate with TNF activation in patients (132) with advanced HIV infection. The TNF family molecule RANKL and its receptor have also been recognized as important regulators of bone remodeling and have been suggested to be an important mechanism in the development of osteoporosis and osteopenia in HIV (122).

Other factors that have been associated with decreased BMD in HIV-infected individuals include duration of HIV infection and low BMI, history of weight loss, previous use of corticosteroids, hypogonadism, physical inactivity, and smoking, all of which are all common in HIV-infected individuals (118,125,128,133). HIV-infected postmenopausal women also have increased bone loss compared with HIV-uninfected postmenopausal women, suggesting that the combination of HIV infection and menopause may worsen bone loss (129). Another study also demonstrated that androgen deficiency, which occurs with aging, is associated with an increased prevalence of osteopenia and osteoporosis (134). Whether the loss of androgen is directly associated with bone loss or mediated through loss of lean mass is unclear.

The value of routine screening with DXA scans to prevent or manage osteoporosis and osteopenia in HIV-infected individuals remains unclear. As part of the management for osteopenia or osteoporosis, adequate intake of calcium and vitamin D, exercise, cessation of smoking, and decrease in alcohol consumption should be encouraged. Several longitudinal studies in HIV-infected individuals have demonstrated the safety and efficacy of bisphosphonates in the therapy of osteopenia and osteoporosis (135–137). Therefore, HIV-infected patients with osteopenia, osteoporosis, or established fractures should be offered bisphosphonates along with calcium and vitamin D supplementation.

Osteonecrosis, or "avascular necrosis," refers to ischemia or infarction of the cellular constituents of the bone and usually involves the hip, but has also been reported in the shoulder, knee, and ankle in HIV-infected individuals. Osteonecrosis was first described in 1990 during the pre-HAART era (138), and some have suggested an increasing incidence in the HAART era (139,140). The prevalence of osteonecrosis has been reported in 4.4% in one study that performed MRI of the hip in 339 HIV-infected patients (141). That study later demonstrated an incidence in HIV-infected individuals that was about 100 times higher than the annual incidence of approximately 0.003 to 0.006 cases per 100 person-years in the general population (142). However, it remains unclear if the increased incidence is a result of a direct effect of the antiretroviral drugs.

Risk factors for osteonecrosis include corticosteroid use (including short courses as part of treatment for *Pneumocystis jiroveci* pneumonia), hypercoagulable states such as antiphospholipid syndrome and alcohol and tobacco use, use of megace or testosterone, and hyperlipidemia (143,144). Some researchers have suggested that the possible increase in osteonecrosis in the HAART era may be due to the increase in hyperlipidemia associated with PI use and not a direct effect of the antiretroviral drugs.

Patients with osteonecrosis, particularly of the hip, usually present with hip pain. MRI is currently the preferred imaging modality to evaluate an HIV-infected patient with hip pain and suspected osteonecrosis. Management is generally conservative, although total hip replacement is not uncommon.

REFERENCES

1. Schackman BR, Gebo KA, Walensky RP, et al. The lifetime cost of current human immunodeficiency virus care in the United States. Med Care 2006; 44(11):990–997.
2. Carr A, Samaras K, Burton S, et al. A syndrome of peripheral lipodystrophy, hyperlipidaemia and insulin resistance in patients receiving HIV protease inhibitors. AIDS 1998; 12(7):F51–F58.
3. Lo JC, Mulligan K, Tai VW, et al. "Buffalo hump" in men with HIV-1 infection. Lancet 1998; 351(9106):867–870.
4. Miller KD, Jones E, Yanovski JA, et al. Visceral abdominal-fat accumulation associated with use of indinavir. Lancet 1998; 351(9106):871–875.
5. Miller KK, Daly PA, Sentochnik D, et al. Pseudo-Cushing's syndrome in human immunodeficiency virus-infected patients. Clin Infect Dis 1998; 27(1):68–72.
6. Striker R, Conlin D, Marx M, et al. Localized adipose tissue hypertrophy in patients receiving human immunodeficiency virus protease inhibitors. Clin Infect Dis 1998; 27(1):218–220.
7. Dong KL, Bausserman LL, Flynn MM, et al. Changes in body habitus and serum lipid abnormalities in HIV-positive women on highly active antiretroviral therapy (HAART). J Acquir Immune Defic Syndr 1999; 21(2):107–113.
8. Galli M, Veglia F, Angarano G, et al. Gender differences in antiretroviral drug-related adipose tissue alterations. J Acquir Immune Defic Syndr 2003; 34(1):58–61.
9. Gervasoni C, Ridolfo AL, Trifiro G, et al. Redistribution of body fat in HIV-infected women undergoing combined antiretroviral therapy. AIDS 1999; 13(4): 465–471.
10. Herry I, Bernard L, de Truchis P, et al. Hypertrophy of the breasts in a patient treated with indinavir. Clin Infect Dis 1997; 25(4):937–938.
11. FRAM Study Investigators. Fat distribution in men with HIV infection. J Acquir Immune Defic Syndr 2005; 40(2):121–131.
12. Fat distribution in women with HIV infection. J Acquir Immune Defic Syndr 2006; 42(5):562–571.
13. Mulligan K, Anastos K, Justman J, et al. Fat distribution in HIV-infected women in the United States: DEXA substudy in the Women's Interagency HIV Study. J Acquir Immune Defic Syndr 2005; 38(1):18–22.

14. Tien PC, Cole SR, Williams CM, et al. Incidence of lipoatrophy and lipohypertrophy in the women's interagency HIV study. J Acquir Immune Defic Syndr 2003; 34(5):461–466.
15. Brown TT, Chu H, Wang Z, et al. Longitudinal increases in waist circumference are associated with HIV-serostatus, independent of antiretroviral therapy. Aids 2007; 21(13):1731–1738.
16. Mallon P, Miller J, Cooper D, et al. Prospective evaluation of the effects of antiretroviral therapy on body composition in HIV-1 infected men starting therapy. AIDS 2003; 17(7):971–979.
17. Tien PC, Grunfeld C. What is HIV-associated lipodystrophy? Defining fat distribution changes in HIV infection. Curr Opin Infect Dis 2004; 17(1):27–32.
18. Saint-Marc T, Partisani M, Poizot-Martin I, et al. A syndrome of peripheral fat wasting (lipodystrophy) in patients receiving long-term nucleoside analogue therapy. AIDS 1999; 13(13):1659–1667.
19. Carr A, Workman C, Smith DE, et al. Abacavir substitution for nucleoside analogs in patients with HIV lipoatrophy: a randomized trial. Jama 2002; 288(2):207–215.
20. Martin A, Smith DE, Carr A, et al. Reversibility of lipoatrophy in HIV-infected patients 2 years after switching from a thymidine analogue to abacavir: the MITOX Extension Study. Aids 2004; 18(7):1029–1036.
21. McComsey GA, Ward DJ, Hessenthaler SM, et al. Improvement in lipoatrophy associated with highly active antiretroviral therapy in human immunodeficiency virus-infected patients switched from stavudine to abacavir or zidovudine: the results of the TARHEEL study. Clin Infect Dis 2004; 38(2):263–270.
22. Moyle G, Sabin C, Cartledge J, et al. A 48-week, randomized, open-label comparative study of tenofovir DF vs. abacavir as substitutes for a thymidine analog in persons with lipoatrophy and sustained virologic suppression on HAART. In: Health FfRaH, ed. 12th Conference on Retroviruses and Opportunistic Infections. Boston, MA, 2005.
23. Tien PC, Schneider MF, Cole SR, et al. Relation of Stavudine Discontinuation to Anthropometric Changes Among HIV-Infected Women. J Acquir Immune Defic Syndr 2007; 44(1):43–48.
24. Moyle GJ, Baldwin C, Langroudi B, et al. A 48-week, randomized, open-label comparison of three abacavir-based substitution approaches in the management of dyslipidemia and peripheral lipoatrophy. J Acquir Immune Defic Syndr 2003; 33(1):22–28.
25. Ruiz L, Negredo E, Domingo P, et al. Antiretroviral treatment simplification with nevirapine in protease inhibitor-experienced patients with HIV-associated lipodystrophy: 1-year prospective follow-up of a multicenter, randomized, controlled study. J Acquir Immune Defic Syndr 2001; 27(3):229–236.
26. Kakuda TN. Pharmacology of nucleoside and nucleotide reverse transcriptase inhibitor-induced mitochondrial toxicity. Clin Ther 2000; 22(6):685–708.
27. Walker UA, Bickel M, Lutke Volksbeck SI, et al. Evidence of nucleoside analogue reverse transcriptase inhibitor–associated genetic and structural defects of mitochondria in adipose tissue of HIV-infected patients. J Acquir Immune Defic Syndr 2002; 29(2):117–121.
28. McComsey GA, Paulsen DM, Lonergan JT, et al. Improvements in lipoatrophy, mitochondrial DNA levels and fat apoptosis after replacing stavudine with abacavir or zidovudine. Aids 2005; 19(1):15–23.

29. van Wijk JP, de Koning EJ, Cabezas MC, et al. Comparison of rosiglitazone and metformin for treating HIV lipodystrophy: a randomized trial. Ann Intern Med 2005; 143(5):337–346.

30. Carr A, Workman C, Carey D, et al. No effect of rosiglitazone for treatment of HIV-1 lipoatrophy: randomised, double-blind, placebo-controlled trial. Lancet 2004; 363(9407):429–438.

31. Cavalcanti RB, Raboud J, Shen S, et al. A randomized, placebo-controlled trial of rosiglitazone for HIV-related lipoatrophy. J Infect Dis 2007; 195(12):1754–1761.

32. Hadigan C, Yawetz S, Thomas A, et al. Metabolic effects of rosiglitazone in HIV lipodystrophy: a randomized, controlled trial. Ann Intern Med 2004; 140(10): 786–794.

33. Mallon PW, Miller J, Kovacic JC, et al. Effect of pravastatin on body composition and markers of cardiovascular disease in HIV-infected men—a randomized, placebo-controlled study. AIDS 2006; 20(7):1003–1010.

34. McComsey GA, O'Riordan M, Setzer B, et al. Uridine supplementation in HIV lipoatrophy: pilot trial on safety and effect on mitochondrial indices. Eur J Clin Nutr 2007.

35. Moyle GJ, Lysakova L, Brown S, et al. A randomized open-label study of imme-diate versus delayed polylactic acid injections for the cosmetic management of facial lipoatrophy in persons with HIV infection. HIV Med 2004; 5(2):82–87.

36. Valantin MA, Aubron-Olivier C, Ghosn J, et al. Polylactic acid implants (New-Fill) to correct facial lipoatrophy in HIV-infected patients: results of the open-label study VEGA. Aids 2003; 17(17):2471–2477.

37. Heath K, Hogg R, Singer J, Chan K, et al. Antiretroviral treatment patterns and incident HIV-associated morphologic and lipid abnormalities in a population-based cohort. J Acquir Immune Defic Syndr 2002; 30:440–447.

38. Lichtenstein KA, Ward DJ, Moorman AC, et al. Clinical assessment of HIV-associated lipodystrophy in an ambulatory population. Aids 2001; 15(11):1389–1398.

39. Saves M, Raffi F, Capeau J, et al. Factors related to lipodystrophy and metabolic alterations in patients with human immunodeficiency virus infection receiving highly active antiretroviral therapy. Clin Infect Dis 2002; 34:1397–1405.

40. Hommes MJ, Romijn JA, Endert E, et al. Insulin sensitivity and insulin clearance in human immunodeficiency virus-infected men. Metabolism 1991; 40(6):651–656.

41. Walli R, Goebel FD, Demant T. Impaired glucose tolerance and protease inhibitors. Ann Intern Med 1998; 129(10):837–838.

42. Brar I, Shuter J, Thomas A, et al. A comparison of factors associated with prevalent diabetes mellitus among HIV-Infected antiretroviral-naive individuals versus indi-viduals in the National Health and Nutritional Examination Survey cohort. J Acquir Immune Defic Syndr 2007; 45(1):66–71.

43. Behrens G, Dejam A, Schmidt H, et al. Impaired glucose tolerance, beta cell function and lipid metabolism in HIV patients under treatment with protease inhibitors. AIDS 1999; 13(10):F63–F70.

44. Dube MP, Johnson DL, Currier JS, et al. Protease inhibitor-associated hyper-glycaemia. Lancet 1997; 350(9079):713–714.

45. Mulligan K, Grunfeld C, Tai VW, et al. Hyperlipidemia and insulin resistance are induced by protease inhibitors independent of changes in body composition in patients with HIV infection. J Acquir Immune Defic Syndr 2000; 23(1):35–43.

46. Murata H, Hruz PW, Mueckler M. The mechanism of insulin resistance caused by HIV protease inhibitor therapy. J Biol Chem 2000; 275(27):20251–20254.

47. Noor MA, Seneviratne T, Aweeka FT, et al. Indinavir acutely inhibits insulin-stimulated glucose disposal in humans: a randomized, placebo-controlled study. AIDS 2002; 16(5):F1–F8.

48. Lee GA, Lo JC, Aweeka F, et al. Single-dose lopinavir-ritonavir acutely inhibits insulin-mediated glucose disposal in healthy volunteers. Clin Infect Dis 2006; 43(5): 658–660.

49. Lee GA, Seneviratne T, Noor MA, et al. The metabolic effects of lopinavir/ritonavir in HIV-negative men. AIDS 2004; 18(4):641–649.

50. Noor MA, Lo JC, Mulligan K, et al. Metabolic effects of indinavir in healthy HIV-seronegative men. AIDS 2001; 15(7):F11–F8.

51. Shlay JC, Bartsch G, Peng G, et al. Long-term body composition and metabolic changes in antiretroviral naive persons randomized to protease inhibitor-, non-nucleoside reverse transcriptase inhibitor-, or protease inhibitor plus nonnucleoside reverse transcriptase inhibitor-based strategy. J Acquir Immune Defic Syndr 2007; 44(5):506–517.

52. Brown TT, Li X, Cole SR, et al. Cumulative exposure to nucleoside analogue reverse transcriptase inhibitors is associated with insulin resistance markers in the Multicenter AIDS Cohort Study. AIDS 2005; 19(13):1375–1383.

53. Tien PC, Schneider MF, Cole SR, et al. Antiretroviral therapy exposure and incidence of diabetes mellitus in the Women's Interagency HIV Study. AIDS 2007; 21(13):1739–1745.

54. Howard AA, Floris-Moore M, Arnsten JH, et al. Disorders of glucose metabolism among HIV-infected women. Clin Infect Dis 2005; 40(10):1492–1499.

55. Howard AA, Floris-Moore M, Lo Y, et al. Abnormal glucose metabolism among older men with or at risk of HIV infection. HIV Med 2006; 7(6):389–396.

56. Grunfeld C, Rimland D, Gibert CL, et al. Association of Upper Trunk and Visceral Adipose Tissue. J Acquir Immune Defic Syndr 2007; Publish Ahead of Print.

57. Hadigan C, Miller K, Corcoran C, et al. Fasting hyperinsulinemia and changes in regional body composition in human immunodeficiency virus-infected women. J Clin Endocrinol Metab 1999; 84(6):1932–1937.

58. Chen Z, Bassford T, Green SB, et al. Postmenopausal hormone therapy and body composition–a substudy of the estrogen plus progestin trial of the Women's Health Initiative. Am J Clin Nutr 2005; 82(3):651–656.

59. Haffner SM, Karhapaa P, Mykkanen L, et al. Insulin resistance, body fat distribution, and sex hormones in men. Diabetes 1994; 43(2):212–219.

60. Huang JS, Wilkie SJ, Dolan S, et al. Reduced testosterone levels in human immunodeficiency virus-infected women with weight loss and low weight. Clin Infect Dis 2003; 36(4):499–506.

61. Ding EL, Song Y, Malik VS, et al. Sex differences of endogenous sex hormones and risk of type 2 diabetes: a systematic review and meta-analysis. JAMA 2006; 295 (11): 1288–1299.

62. Muller M, Aleman A, Grobbee DE, et al. Endogenous sex hormone levels and cognitive function in aging men: is there an optimal level? Neurology 2005; 64(5): 866–871.

63. Harman SM. Testosterone in older men after the Institute of Medicine Report: where do we go from here? Climacteric 2005; 8(2):124–135.

64. Dube MP, Parker RA, Mulligan K, et al. Effects of potent antiretroviral therapy on free testosterone levels and fat-free mass in men in a prospective, randomized trial: A5005s, a substudy of AIDS Clinical Trials Group Study 384. Clin Infect Dis 2007; 45(1):120–126.

65. Wunder DM, Bersinger NA, Fux CA, et al. Hypogonadism in HIV-1-infected men is common and does not resolve during antiretroviral therapy. Antivir Ther 2007; 12(2):261–265.

66. Wisniewski AB, Brown TT, John M, et al. Hypothalamic-pituitary-gonadal function in men and women using heroin and cocaine, stratified by HIV status. Gend Med 2007; 4(1):35–44.

67. Crum NF, Furtek KJ, Olson PE, et al. A review of hypogonadism and erectile dysfunction among HIV-infected men during the pre- and post-HAART eras: diagnosis, pathogenesis, and management. AIDS Patient Care STDS 2005; 19(10): 655–671.

68. Crum-Cianflone NF, Bavaro M, Hale B, et al. Erectile dysfunction and hypogonadism among men with HIV. AIDS Patient Care STDS 2007; 21(1):9–19.

69. Montano M, Flanagan JN, Jiang L, et al. Transcriptional profiling of testosterone-regulated genes in the skeletal muscle of human immunodeficiency virus-infected men experiencing weight loss. J Clin Endocrinol Metab 2007; 92(7):2793–2802.

70. Bhasin S, Parker RA, Sattler F, et al. Effects of testosterone supplementation on whole body and regional fat mass and distribution in human immunodeficiency virus-infected men with abdominal obesity. J Clin Endocrinol Metab 2007; 92(3): 1049–1057.

71. Behler C, Shade S, Gregory K, et al. Anemia and HIV in the antiretroviral era: potential significance of testosterone. AIDS Res Hum Retroviruses 2005; 21(3): 200–206.

72. Aragon-Ching JB, Williams KM, Gulley JL. Impact of androgen-deprivation therapy on the immune system: implications for combination therapy of prostate cancer. Front Biosci 2007; 12:4957–4971.

73. Barbee RA, Hicks MJ, Grosso D, et al. The maternal immune response in coccidioidomycosis. Is pregnancy a risk factor for serious infection? Chest 1991; 100(3): 709–715.

74. Boyd AS, Morris LF, Phillips CM, et al. Psoriasis and pregnancy: hormone and immune system interaction. Int J Dermatol 1996; 35(3):169–172.

75. Cohen P. Sex and shedding of human immunodeficiency virus. J Infect Dis 2000; 182(1):375–376.

76. Diwan VK, Thorson A. Sex, gender, and tuberculosis. Lancet 1999; 353(9157): 1000–1001.

77. Jansson L, Holmdahl R. Estrogen-mediated immunosuppression in autoimmune diseases. Inflamm Res 1998; 47(7):290–301.

78. Kaushic C, Murdin AD, Underdown BJ, et al. Chlamydia trachomatis infection in the female reproductive tract of the rat: influence of progesterone on infectivity and immune response. Infect Immun 1998; 66(3):893–898.

79. Kaushic C, Zhou F, Murdin AD, et al. Effects of estradiol and progesterone on susceptibility and early immune responses to Chlamydia trachomatis infection in the female reproductive tract. Infect Immun 2000; 68(7):4207–4216.

80. Klein S. Host factors mediating sex differences in viral infection. Gend Med 2005; 2(4):197–207.

81. Taylor RN, Greenblatt RM. Sex and sheddingof human immunodeficiency virus. J Infect Dis 2000; 182(1):376.
82. Wilder RL. Adrenal and gonadal steroid hormone deficiency in the pathogenesis of rheumatoid arthritis. J Rheumatol Suppl 1996; 44:10–12.
83. Beagley KW, Gockel CM. Regulation of innate and adaptive immunity by the female sex hormones oestradiol and progesterone. FEMS Immunol Med Microbiol 2003; 38(1):13–22.
84. Greenblatt RM, Ameli N, Grant RM, et al. Impact of the ovulatory cycle on virologic and immunologic markers in HIV-infected women. J Infect Dis 2000; 181(1):82–90.
85. Long EM, Martin HL Jr., Kreiss JK, et al. Gender differences in HIV-1 diversity at time of infection. Nat Med 2000; 6(1):71–75.
86. Cu-Uvin S. Effect of the menstrual cycle on virological parameters. J Acquir Immune Defic Syndr 2005; 38 Suppl 1:S33–S34.
87. Athreya BH, Pletcher J, Zulian F, et al. Subset-specific effects of sex hormones and pituitary gonadotropins on human lymphocyte proliferation in vitro. Clin Immunol Immunopathol 1993; 66(3):201–211.
88. Giglio T, Imro MA, Filaci G, et al. Immune cell circulating subsets are affected by gonadal function. Life Sci 1994; 54(18):1305–1312.
89. Kiess W, Liu LL, Hall NR. Lymphocyte subset distribution and natural killer cell activity in men with idiopathic hypogonadotropic hypogonadism. Acta Endocrinol (Copenh) 1991; 124(4):399–404.
90. Mathur S, Mathur RS, Goust JM, et al. Cyclic variations in white cell subpopulations in the human menstrual cycle: correlations with progesterone and estradiol. Clin Immunol Immunopathol 1979; 13(3):246–253.
91. Mylvaganam R, Ahn YS, Harrington WJ, et al. Differences in T cell subsets between men and women with idiopathic thrombocytopenic purpura. Blood 1985; 66(4): 967–972.
92. Rodrigues A, Fischer TK, Valentiner-Branth P, et al. Community cohort study of rotavirus and other enteropathogens: are routine vaccinations associated with sex-differential incidence rates? Vaccine 2006; 24(22):4737–4746.
93. van Benthem BH, Vernazza P, Coutinho RA, et al. The impact of pregnancy and menopause on CD4 lymphocyte counts in HIV-infected women. AIDS 2002; 16(6): 919–924.
94. Clark RA, Mulligan K, Stamenovic E, et al. Frequency of anovulation and early menopause among women enrolled in selected adult AIDS clinical trials group studies. J Infect Dis 2001; 184(10):1325–1327.
95. Fantry LE, Zhan M, Taylor GH, et al. Age of menopause and menopausal symptoms in HIV-infected women. AIDS Patient Care STDS 2005; 19(11):703–711.
96. Miller SA, Santoro N, Lo Y, et al. Menopause symptoms in HIV-infected and drug-using women. Menopause 2005; 12(3):348–356.
97. Schoenbaum EE, Hartel D, Lo Y, et al. HIV infection, drug use, and onset of natural menopause. Clin Infect Dis 2005; 41(10):1517–1524.
98. Cejtin HE, Kalinowski A, Bacchetti P, et al. Effects of human immunodeficiency virus on protracted amenorrhea and ovarian dysfunction. Obstet Gynecol 2006; 108(6):1423–1431.

99. Ferreira CE, Pinto-Neto AM, Conde DM, et al. Menopause symptoms in women infected with HIV: prevalence and associated factors. Gynecol Endocrinol 2007; 23(4):198–205.
100. Herbst KL, Calof OM, Hsia SH, et al. Effects of transdermal testosterone administration on insulin sensitivity, fat mass and distribution, and markers of inflammation and thrombolysis in human immunodeficiency virus-infected women with mild to moderate weight loss. Fertil Steril 2006; 85(6):1794–1802.
101. Madge S, Smith CJ, Lampe FC, et al. No association between HIV disease and its treatment and thyroid function. HIV Med 2007; 8(1):22–27.
102. Hoffmann CJ, Brown TT. Thyroid function abnormalities in HIV-infected patients. Clin Infect Dis 2007; 45(4):488–494.
103. Kaw YT, Brunnemer C. Initial diagnosis of disseminated cryptococcosis and acquired immunodeficiency syndrome by fine needle aspiration of the thyroid. A case report. Acta Cytol 1994; 38(3):427–430.
104. Keyhani-Rofagha S, Piquero C. Pneumocystis carinii thyroiditis diagnosis by fine needle aspiration cytology: a case report. Acta Cytol 1996; 40(2):307–310.
105. Kiertiburanakul S, Sungkanuparph S, Malathum K, et al. Concomitant tuberculous and cryptococcal thyroid abscess in a human immunodeficiency virus-infected patient. Scand J Infect Dis 2003; 35(1):68–70.
106. Martin-Davila P, Quereda C, Rodriguez H, et al. Thyroid abscess due to Rhodococcus equi in a patient infected with the human immunodeficiency virus. Eur J Clin Microbiol Infect Dis 1998; 17(1):55–57.
107. Price P, Mathiot N, Krueger R, et al. Immune dysfunction and immune restoration disease in HIV patients given highly active antiretroviral therapy. J Clin Virol 2001; 22(3):279–287.
108. Chen F, Day SL, Metcalfe RA, et al. Characteristics of autoimmune thyroid disease occurring as a late complication of immune reconstitution in patients with advanced human immunodeficiency virus (HIV) disease. Medicine (Baltimore) 2005; 84(2):98–106.
109. Jubault V, Penfornis A, Schillo F, et al. Sequential occurrence of thyroid autoantibodies and Graves' disease after immune restoration in severely immunocompromised human immunodeficiency virus-1-infected patients. J Clin Endocrinol Metab 2000; 85(11):4254–4257.
110. Knysz B, Bolanowski M, Klimczak M, et al. Graves' disease as an immune reconstitution syndrome in an HIV-1-positive patient commencing effective antiretroviral therapy: case report and literature review. Viral Immunol 2006; 19(1):102–107.
111. Beltran S, Lescure FX, El Esper I, et al. Subclinical hypothyroidism in HIV-infected patients is not an autoimmune disease. Horm Res 2006; 66(1):21–26.
112. Wong KH, Chow WS, Lee SS. Clinical hyperthyroidism in Chinese patients with stable HIV disease. Clin Infect Dis 2004; 39(8):1257–1259.
113. Collazos J, Ibarra S, Mayo J. Thyroid hormones in HIV-infected patients in the highly active antiretroviral therapy era: evidence of an interrelation between the thyroid axis and the immune system. AIDS 2003; 17(5):763–765.
114. Madeddu G, Spanu A, Chessa F, et al. Thyroid function in human immunodeficiency virus patients treated with highly active antiretroviral therapy (HAART): a longitudinal study. Clin Endocrinol (Oxf) 2006; 64(4):375–383.

115. Ladenson PW, Singer PA, Ain KB, et al. American Thyroid Association guidelines for detection of thyroid dysfunction. Arch Intern Med 2000; 160(11):1573–1575.
116. Brown TT, Qaqish RB. Antiretroviral therapy and the prevalence of osteopenia and osteoporosis: a meta-analytic review. AIDS 2006; 20(17):2165–2174.
117. Madeddu G, Spanu A, Solinas P, et al. Bone mass loss and vitamin D metabolism impairment in HIV patients receiving highly active antiretroviral therapy. Q J Nucl Med Mol Imaging 2004; 48(1):39–48.
118. Nolan D, Upton R, McKinnon E, et al. Stable or increasing bone mineral density in HIV-infected patients treated with nelfinavir or indinavir. AIDS 2001; 15(10): 1275–1280.
119. Tebas P, Powderly WG, Claxton S, et al. Accelerated bone mineral loss in HIV-infected patients receiving potent antiretroviral therapy. Aids 2000; 14(4):F63–F67.
120. Amiel C, Ostertag A, Slama L, et al. BMD is reduced in HIV-infected men irrespective of treatment. J Bone Miner Res 2004; 19(3):402–409.
121. Bruera D, Luna N, David DO, et al. Decreased bone mineral density in HIV-infected patients is independent of antiretroviral therapy. AIDS 2003; 17(13):1917–1923.
122. Konishi M, Takahashi K, Yoshimoto E, et al. Association between osteopenia/osteoporosis and the serum RANKL in HIV-infected patients. AIDS 2005; 19(11): 1240–1241.
123. Dube MP, Qian D, Edmondson-Melancon H, et al. Prospective, intensive study of metabolic changes associated with 48 weeks of amprenavir-based antiretroviral therapy. Clin Infect Dis 2002; 35(4):475–481.
124. Fernandez-Rivera J, Garcia R, Lozano F, et al. Relationship between low bone mineral density and highly active antiretroviral therapy including protease inhibitors in HIV-infected patients. HIV Clin Trials 2003; 4(5):337–346.
125. Mondy K, Yarasheski K, Powderly WG, et al. Longitudinal evolution of bone mineral density and bone markers in human immunodeficiency virus-infected individuals. Clin Infect Dis 2003; 36(4):482–490.
126. Gallant JE, Staszewski S, Pozniak AL, et al. Efficacy and safety of tenofovir DF vs stavudine in combination therapy in antiretroviral-naive patients: a 3-year randomized trial. JAMA 2004; 292(2):191–201.
127. Brown TT, Ruppe MD, Kassner R, et al. Reduced bone mineral density in human immunodeficiency virus-infected patients and its association with increased central adiposity and postload hyperglycemia. J Clin Endocrinol Metab 2004; 89(3): 1200–1206.
128. Dolan SE, Huang JS, Killilea KM, et al. Reduced bone density in HIV-infected women. AIDS 2004; 18(3):475–483.
129. Yin M, Dobkin J, Brudney K, et al. Bone mass and mineral metabolism in HIV+ postmenopausal women. Osteoporos Int 2005; 16(11):1345–1352.
130. Amorosa V, Tebas P. Bone disease and HIV infection. Clin Infect Dis 2006; 42(1): 108–14.
131. Hittinger G, Poggi C, Delbeke E, et al. Correlation between plasma levels of cytokines and HIV-1 RNA copy number in HIV-infected patients. Infection 1998; 26(2):100–103.
132. Aukrust P, Haug CJ, Ueland T, et al. Decreased bone formative and enhanced resorptive markers in human immunodeficiency virus infection: indication of normalization of the bone-remodeling process during highly active antiretroviral therapy. J Clin Endocrinol Metab 1999; 84(1):145–150.

133. Arnsten JH, Freeman R, Howard AA, et al. Decreased bone mineral density and increased fracture risk in aging men with or at risk for HIV infection. AIDS 2007; 21(5):617–623.
134. Dolan SE, Carpenter S, Grinspoon S. Effects of weight, body composition, and testosterone on bone mineral density in HIV-infected women. J Acquir Immune Defic Syndr 2007; 45(2):161–167.
135. Guaraldi G, Orlando G, Madeddu G, et al. Alendronate reduces bone resorption in HIV-associated osteopenia/osteoporosis. HIV Clin Trials 2004; 5(5):269–277.
136. Mondy K, Powderly WG, Claxton SA, et al. Alendronate, vitamin D, and calcium for the treatment of osteopenia/osteoporosis associated with HIV infection. J Acquir Immune Defic Syndr 2005; 38(4):426–431.
137. Negredo E, Martinez-Lopez E, Paredes R, et al. Reversal of HIV-1-associated osteoporosis with once-weekly alendronate. AIDS 2005; 19(3):343–345.
138. Goorney BP, Lacey H, Thurairajasingam S, et al. Avascular necrosis of the hip in a man with HIV infection. Genitourin Med 1990; 66(6):451–452.
139. Gutierrez F, Padilla S, Ortega E, et al. Avascular necrosis of the bone in HIV-infected patients: incidence and associated factors. AIDS 2002; 16(3):481–483.
140. Keruly JC, Chaisson RE, Moore RD. Increasing incidence of avascular necrosis of the hip in HIV-infected patients. J Acquir Immune Defic Syndr 2001; 28(1):101–102.
141. Miller KD, Masur H, Jones EC, et al. High prevalence of osteonecrosis of the femoral head in HIV-infected adults. Ann Intern Med 2002; 137(1):17–25.
142. Morse CG, Mican JM, Jones EC, et al. The incidence and natural history of osteonecrosis in HIV-infected adults. Clin Infect Dis 2007; 44(5):739–748.
143. Glesby MJ, Hoover DR, Vaamonde CM. Osteonecrosis in patients infected with human immunodeficiency virus: a case-control study. J Infect Dis 2001; 184(4):519–523.
144. Mary-Krause M, Billaud E, Poizot-Martin I, et al. Risk factors for osteonecrosis in HIV-infected patients: impact of treatment with combination antiretroviral therapy. AIDS 2006; 20(12):1627–1635.

6

The Renal System

Christina M. Wyatt

*Division of Nephrology, Mount Sinai School of Medicine,
New York, New York, U.S.A.*

INTRODUCTION

Kidney disease has been recognized as a complication of HIV and AIDS since the early 1980s (1). Renal function is known to diminish with age (2,3). Thus, both acute and chronic kidney disease are likely to present an increasing burden on the aging population of antiretroviral-treated patients. Projected increases in the prevalence of end-stage renal disease attributed to HIV (4) are compounded by racial disparities in new HIV/AIDS diagnoses among older adults, as minority patients at increased risk for kidney disease make up a growing proportion of the aging HIV population. Even in the absence of kidney disease or systemic illness, kidney function declines slowly with age (5). Recognition of this physiologic, age-related decline in kidney function is essential to guide medication dosing and identify patients at increased risk of acute renal failure, medication toxicity, and chronic kidney disease.

ACUTE RENAL FAILURE IN HIV

Acute renal failure is an increasingly important complication of HIV in the aging cohort of antiretroviral-treated patients. In addition to older age, other risk factors for acute renal failure include underlying chronic kidney disease, advanced HIV infection or AIDS, and hepatitis C coinfection (6,7). Common causes of acute renal failure are similar to those observed before the introduction of antiretroviral therapy, including volume depletion, sepsis, and medication toxicity (6). End-stage liver disease is also an increasingly common cause of acute renal failure in the aging cohort of patients with hepatitis virus coinfection (6). Recognition of acute renal failure should prompt careful review of all medications to identify potential nephrotoxins, as well as any medications requiring dose adjustment.

MEDICATION NEPHROTOXICITY

Protease Inhibitors

The first antiretroviral agent to demonstrate significant nephrotoxicity was the protease inhibitor indinavir (8–11), which has been associated with obstructive nephropathy and chronic interstitial nephritis (Table 1). As the only protease inhibitor that undergoes clinically significant renal elimination, indinavir is poorly soluble at physiologic urine pH. Subclinical crystalluria has been observed in up to two-thirds of indinavir-treated patients, with symptomatic disease in 8% of indinavir-treated patients in one cohort (9). Obstructive nephropathy may respond to hydration and discontinuation of the drug, and guidelines recommend maintaining high urine flow rates (12). More recently, the protease inhibitor atazanavir has also been associated with nephrolithiasis and obstructive nephropathy, although the incidence appears to be much lower than with indinavir (13). Saquinavir and nelfinavir have each been associated with a single report of nephrolithiasis (14,15).

The protease inhibitor ritonavir has been associated with rare cases of acute renal failure (16,17) and has been reported to potentiate the nephrotoxicity

Table 1 Potential Nephrotoxicity of Antiretroviral Therapy

Antiretroviral class	Specific antiretroviral	Reported nephrotoxicity
Nucleoside	Didanosine	Type B lactic acidosis
		Isolated cases of acute renal failure
	Stavudine	Type B lactic acidosis
	Other nucleosides	Rare cases of lactic acidosis
Nucleotide	Tenofovir	Proximal tubular toxicity
		Acute renal failure
		Decline in kidney function
Non-nucleoside	Efavirenz/nevirapine	Rare involvement of the kidney in systemic hypersensitivity reactions
Protease inhibitor	Atazanavir	Nephrolithiasis
	Indinavir	Crystal nephropathy
	Ritonavir	Acute renal failure
	Other protease inhibitors	Isolated reports of nephrolithiasis
Fusion inhibitor	Enfurvitide	Single report of glomerulonephritis

of indinavir and tenofovir (18). Although ritonavir inhibits several tubular transport proteins in vitro, it does not interfere with the multidrug resistance protein-4 (MRP4) efflux pump responsible for the removal of tenofovir from tubular epithelial cells (19). Until further studies clarify the nature of the potential drug interaction, patients receiving combination therapy with ritonavir and tenofovir or indinavir should be monitored for toxicity.

Nucleoside Reverse Transcriptase Inhibitors

The nucleoside analogues have been associated with mitochondrial dysfunction and Type B lactic acidosis (20). While nucleoside analogues are only rarely associated with proximal tubular toxicity (21), nucleoside-induced mitochondrial dysfunction has been hypothesized to potentiate the tubular toxicity of nucleotide analogues (22).

Nucleotide Reverse Transcriptase Inhibitors

Proximal tubular injury was the dose-limiting toxicity associated with the nucleotide analogues cidofovir and adefovir in early clinical trials (23,24). Despite toxicity in animal models, the newer nucleotide reverse transcriptase inhibitor tenofovir was not associated with significant nephrotoxicity in premarketing clinical studies (25–27). With the widespread use of tenofovir in clinical practice, however, this agent has also been associated with proximal tubular injury, nephrogenic diabetes insipidus, acute renal failure, and reduced kidney function (28–30). The nucleotides enter tubular epithelial cells via the organic anion transporters OAT1 and OAT3, and intracellular accumulation is cytotoxic in vitro. Tenofovir interacts primarily with the MRP4 efflux pump on the luminal membrane (19).

Postmarketing data from the tenofovir expanded access program are consistent with an incidence of mild nephrotoxicity approaching 2%, with severe nephrotoxicity occurring less commonly (31). Observational data have also suggested a small but statistically significant decline in kidney function with tenofovir treatment, compared with alternative regimens (32). The long-term effects of chronic tenofovir exposure on kidney function are not known. Expert guidelines recommend monitoring for nephrotoxicity at least biannually in tenofovir-treated patients, including estimation of kidney function and screening for proteinuria or glycosuria (12).

Other Antiretroviral Agents

Acute renal failure has been observed rarely in the setting of hypersensitivity reactions to the non-nucleotide reverse transcriptase inhibitors (33,34) and the fusion inhibitor enfurvitide (35). With the rapid pace of drug development and the potential for recognition of new toxicities in the postmarketing period, readers are encouraged to refer to recent review articles and package inserts for additional information on antiretroviral toxicity and dosing. The potential for antiretroviral therapy to promote kidney disease risk factors such as insulin resistance, hyperlipidemia, and hypertension is discussed elsewhere in this book.

Other Antimicrobial Therapy in HIV/AIDS

Antimicrobial agents used to treat opportunistic infections may also be associated with nephrotoxicity. Treatment of cytomegalovirus infections may be complicated by toxicity associated with both cidofovir (23) and foscarnet (36,37). Ganciclovir was also associated with mild nephrotoxicity in a single study (38) but is the preferred anticytomegalovirus agent in patients with kidney disease. Both intravenous acyclovir (39,40) and sulfadiazine (41) have been associated with crystal precipitation and obstruction. Adequate hydration and appropriate dose adjustment for reduced kidney function may reduce the risk of crystal nephropathy associated with these agents (39,40).

The treatment of pneumocystis with trimethoprim-sulfamethoxazole or pentamidine may be associated with elevations in serum creatinine and potassium. Trimethoprim inhibits tubular secretion of creatinine and does not directly influence kidney function (42), although interference with the tubular secretion of potassium can result in clinically relevant hyperkalemia (43,44). Unlike trimethoprim, the increase in serum creatinine observed with pentamidine is associated with decreased kidney function (45,46). Pentamidine may cause significant hyperkalemia as a result of both reduced kidney function and inhibition of potassium secretion (47).

Antifungal and antibacterial agents may also be associated with nephrotoxicity in patients with HIV. Well-known risk factors for amphotericin toxicity, including cumulative dose, critical illness, and concomitant nephrotoxins (48,49), may also predict the development of nephrotoxicity with other agents such as aminoglycoside antibiotics. Beta-lactam antibiotics and sulfonamides are classically associated with interstitial nephritis, which may not always be accompanied by systemic signs of an allergic reaction (50).

CHRONIC KIDNEY DISEASE IN HIV

The epidemiology of chronic kidney disease among HIV-infected patients is highly dependent on the demographics of the population studied, with a greater burden of kidney disease in minority populations. Prevalence estimates in antiretroviral-treated populations range from less than 5% in the largely Caucasian EuroSIDA cohort (51) to as high as 30% in an urban New York clinic (52). The prevalence of chronic kidney disease increases with age (51,52) and may also be associated with advanced HIV infection and hepatitis C coinfection (52).

SPECIFIC KIDNEY DISEASES IN HIV

The spectrum of kidney disease in patients with HIV includes several HIV-related kidney diseases, as well as an increasing burden of comorbid kidney disease in the aging cohort of antiretroviral-treated patients. Because of overlapping clinical presentations, kidney biopsy is often required for definitive diagnosis.

HIV-Associated Nephropathy

HIV-associated nephropathy (HIVAN) was first described in 1984 (1) and remains the classic kidney disease of HIV infection. In the absence of treatment, HIVAN is a rapidly progressive disease characterized by moderate to severe proteinuria. Kidney biopsy demonstrates collapsing focal segmental glomerulosclerosis and accompanying tubular and interstitial disease. Studies in animal models and cell culture have demonstrated that HIVAN is caused by HIV infection of the kidney (53), consistent with the decreased incidence of HIVAN observed in the era of combination antiretroviral therapy (54). Treatment of HIVAN includes anti-retrovirals and ACE inhibitors or angiotensin receptor blockers, based on observational data and uncontrolled trials. Corticosteroids may be added in patients with significant interstitial inflammation or rapid progression, although the risk of further immunosuppression may outweigh any potential benefit in patients with HIVAN, who typically have advanced HIV or AIDS.

Immune Complex Kidney Disease

HIV infection has also been associated with immune complex kidney diseases, including IgA nephropathy (55) and a unique "lupus-like" glomerulonephritis (56). The clinical presentation may be indistinguishable from HIVAN, although some of the immune complex diseases are characterized by microscopic hematuria in addition to proteinuria. Immune complex kidney diseases appear to be increasingly common (57); however, little is known about the pathogenesis or approach to therapy. In contrast to HIVAN, the role of HIV in the pathogenesis of immune complex kidney disease has not been established, and the benefit of antiretroviral therapy is less clear. Because the hepatitis viruses have also been associated with specific immune complex diseases, in particular membranoproliferative and membranous glomerulonephritis, the diagnosis of immune complex kidney disease should prompt testing for hepatitis virus coinfection. Membranous nephropathy has also been associated with other infections such as syphilis, as well as with solid tumors, and should be considered secondary in HIV patients until underlying infection and malignancy have been excluded.

Comorbid Kidney Disease

In addition to kidney disease associated with HIV or coinfections, aging patients with HIV are increasingly at risk for comorbid kidney disease due to diabetes and hypertension, the leading causes of end-stage renal disease in Western countries. The potential role of HIV and antiretroviral therapy in the development of diabetes and hypertension is discussed elsewhere in this book. The presentation of comorbid kidney disease may also mimic HIVAN or hepatitis-related kidney disease, making kidney biopsy the key to definitive diagnosis in most cases.

RECOGNITION OF KIDNEY DISEASE IN HIV

Regardless of the etiology of kidney disease, early recognition identifies patients who are at increased risk for end-stage renal disease, acute renal failure, and medication toxicity (12,58). Accurate estimation of kidney function is also essential to guide medication dosing, but may be particularly challenging in older patients with HIV.

Estimating Kidney Function

The most commonly used surrogate for kidney function, serum creatinine, is a readily available but insensitive indicator of the glomerular filtration rate (GFR). While creatinine is freely filtered at the glomerulus, the serum creatinine measurement is also influenced by active tubular secretion and by the production of creatinine from skeletal muscle. Aging and chronic disease are often associated with a loss of lean muscle mass and a subsequent decrease in creatinine production, which may mask early decreases in kidney function. Estimation equations such as the Cockcroft–Gault (59) and Modification of Diet in Renal Disease (MDRD) equations (60) adjust for the impact of demographic and anthropomorphic factors on the relationship between serum creatinine and GFR.

These creatinine-based estimation equations were derived in different patient populations using different gold standard measures of GFR. A general understanding of these differences provides some insight into the potential limitations of each formula. The Cockcroft–Gault equation was derived in 249 hospitalized men as an alternative to 24-hour urine creatinine clearance and has since been validated as an estimate of GFR (59). The MDRD equation was derived and validated in over 1,600 men and women with chronic kidney disease using ^{25}I-iothalamate clearance as the gold standard measure (60). Although both equations incorporate data on gender and age, it is notable that the Cockcroft–Gault derivation sample included no women, while the MDRD study excluded patients older than 70 years. In addition, both equations were derived in convenience samples of patients with acute illness or chronic kidney disease, which may explain the decreased precision of these estimates in patients with normal kidney function (61). Finally, neither equation has been well validated in patients with AIDS or other relevant conditions such as cachexia, cirrhosis, and acute renal failure.

Despite the limitations of current estimating equations, creatinine-based GFR estimates are more sensitive than serum creatinine alone. Automated reporting of estimated GFR by clinical laboratories may increase the recognition of kidney disease (62), but does not eliminate the need for careful interpretation by providers. In addition, GFR estimates tend to overestimate true GFR in the normal range, and many laboratories report numerical values only for estimates below 60 mL/min/m^2. The FDA continues to require pharmacokinetic data based on Cockcroft–Gault creatinine clearance so that it may be prudent to base drug dosing decisions on the Cockcroft–Gault estimate in patients with borderline kidney function. Rarely, it will be necessary to select an alternative GFR measurement in situations where surrogate markers of lean muscle mass are likely to be inaccurate, such as in advanced age, obesity, cachexia, cirrhosis, or severe lipodystrophy. Although 24-hour urine creatinine clearance is inexpensive and may provide additional information in patients at extremes of weight, patient education and compliance are central to the validity of the results. More costly direct measures of GFR by radionuclide or radiocontrast clearance should be reserved for patients with discrepant GFR estimates in whom a precise measure of GFR is necessary, and further studies are needed to determine the clinical utility of novel serum markers such as cystatin-c.

Proteinuria and Other Evidence of Kidney Injury

Current guidelines for the recognition of kidney disease also include proteinuria and other evidence of kidney injury in the definition of chronic kidney disease (12,58). Specialty guidelines recommend screening for proteinuria in patients at risk for kidney disease (58), including all new patients presenting for HIV care (12). In patients with stable kidney function, a random urine albumin/creatinine or urine protein/creatinine ratio can replace 24-hour urine collection for the quantification of proteinuria (58). Similar to the GFR estimating equations, these ratios assume stable creatinine production and excretion and may not be accurate in the setting of acute renal failure.

In addition to proteinuria, several other urinary and anatomic abnormalities may also indicate kidney injury (58). Persistent microscopic hematuria or sterile pyuria with a negative urological evaluation may be a marker of early glomerular disease. Glycosuria in the setting of normal blood glucose may indicate proximal tubular damage and should prompt a careful review of medications to identify potential tubular toxins. Radiographic findings such as small kidneys, increased echogenicity, cortical thinning, and parenchymal scarring also represent previous injury and chronic kidney disease. Even in patients with preserved GFR, proteinuria and other markers of kidney damage may indicate an increased risk for medication nephrotoxicity, acute renal failure, and progressive kidney disease.

Diagnosis and Classification of Kidney Disease

The diagnosis of kidney disease may be based on a reduction in GFR or evidence of kidney injury (Table 2). In order to standardize nomenclature, current

Table 2   Stage-Specific Management of Chronic Kidney Disease in HIV

Stage	GFR	Kidney damage	Management in HIV
1	≥90	+	Nephrology referral for diagnosis and treatment
			Control hypertension and diabetes if present
2	60–89	+	As above
3	30–59	+/−	As above; consider medication dose adjustment
			Evaluate for anemia and hyperparathyroidism
4	15–29	+/−	As above; discuss options for dialysis and transplant
			Refer for AV fistula if patient prefers hemodialysis
			Kidney transplant evaluation in selected patients
5	<15 (or dialysis)	+/−	As above
			Dialysis/transplantation if indicated

Evidence of kidney damage may include proteinuria, hematuria or sterile pyuria (with a negative urologic evaluation), or anatomic abnormalities.
Abbreviation: GFR, glomerular filtration rate in $mL/min/m^2$.

guidelines consider a reduction in GFR or a marker of kidney injury "chronic" if the abnormality persists for at least three months (58). According to these guidelines, chronic kidney disease is defined by a GFR below 60 $mL/min/m^2$ or evidence of kidney injury. Classification of chronic kidney disease is based on the degree of GFR impairment and the presence of kidney injury, and expert guidelines for the management of chronic kidney disease vary with stage (58).

MANAGEMENT OF CHRONIC KIDNEY DISEASE IN HIV

Delaying Progression and Preventing Complications

Early recognition of chronic kidney disease allows the initiation of treatment to prevent or delay progression and identifies patients at risk for complications. In patients with chronic kidney disease and proteinuria, blockade of the renin-angiotensin-aldosterone system may reduce proteinuria and delay the progression of kidney disease. Control of comorbid hypertension and diabetes may also delay kidney disease progression and help modify the increased cardiovascular risk associated with chronic kidney disease (58,62,63). In addition to these general approaches, some forms of kidney disease may be amenable to specific therapy, highlighting the importance of kidney biopsy for definitive diagnosis. Although the role of antiretroviral therapy in non-HIVAN kidney disease remains uncertain, expert guidelines recommend consideration of antiretroviral therapy in all patients with HIV and chronic kidney disease (12).

Identification of chronic kidney disease should also prompt evaluation and treatment of common complications such as anemia and hyperparathyroidism

(58). The etiology of anemia in patients with HIV infection is often multifactorial, and providers should identify and correct any nutritional or other deficiencies prior to treatment with erythropoietin analogues. Similarly, bone disease and disorders of calcium-phosphorus metabolism may also occur in patients with HIV independent of kidney disease. Osteoporosis and vitamin D deficiency have both been associated with HIV infection (63) and may be exacerbated in the setting of chronic kidney disease.

Medication Dosing

Recognition of acute or chronic kidney disease should also prompt careful review of current medications to ensure appropriate dose adjustment. Medications that undergo complete or partial elimination by the kidney frequently require dose adjustment at GFR levels below 50 to 60 mL/min/m^2. The FDA and the pharmaceutical industry base dosing guidelines on Cockcroft–Gault creatinine clearance, and this GFR estimate should be used to guide medication dosing in most patients. In addition to antiretroviral therapy, this section addresses antihypertensive agents because of their particular relevance in patients with chronic kidney disease.

Antiretroviral Therapy

Among the currently available antiretroviral agents, the majority of nucleoside and nucleotide reverse transcriptase inhibitors are at least partially eliminated by the kidney and, therefore, require dose adjustment in patients with decreased kidney function (Table 3). Zidovudine undergoes significant hepatic metabolism and only requires dose adjustment in patients on dialysis or with a GFR below 10 mL/min/m^2, and abacavir does not require dose adjustment in the setting of kidney disease. Kidney function should be reassessed at least twice annually in patients taking nucleoside or nucleotide analogues requiring dose adjustment for decreased GFR (12).

Currently available non-nucleoside reverse transcriptase inhibitors and protease inhibitors are primarily metabolized by the hepatic cytochrome p450system and do not require dose reduction for decreased kidney function. Although the clinical significance is unknown, metabolites of nevirapine and delavirdine are found in the urine, and pharmacokinetic data are limited in patients with decreased GFR. Current dosing guidelines do not recommend dose reduction of non-nucleoside reverse transcriptase inhibitors in patients with kidney disease, although a supplemental dose of nevirapine is recommended after hemodialysis. Among the protease inhibitors, only indinavir undergoes significant urinary elimination, and these agents do not require dose adjustment for GFR. The fusion inhibitor enfuvirtide and its metabolite undergo plasma catabolism, and dose adjustment is not necessary in the setting of decreased GFR (64).

Table 3 Elimination and Dosing of Antiretroviral Therapy in Chronic Kidney Disease

	Elimination	Dose adjustment in kidney disease
Nucleosides		
Abacavir	Liver	None
Didanosine	Liver/kidney	GFR < 50–60
Emtricitabine	Liver/kidney	GFR < 50–60
Lamivudine	Kidney	GFR < 50–60
Stavudine	Liver/kidney	GFR < 50–60
Zalcitabine	Kidney	GFR < 50–60
Zidovudine	Liver/kidney	GFR < 10
Nucleotides		
Tenofovir	Kidney	GFR < 50–60
Non-nucleosides		
Delavirdine	Liver	None
Efavirenz	Liver	None
Nevirapine	Liver	Extra dose after hemodialysis
Protease inhibitors		
Amprenavir	Liver	None
Atazanavir	Liver	None
Fosamprenavir	Liver	None
Indinavir	Liver/ kidney	None
Lopinavir-ritonavir	Liver	None
Nelfinavir	Liver	None
Ritonavir	Liver	None
Saquinavir	Liver	None
Fusion Inhibitors		
Enfurvitide	Plasma catabolism	None

Abbreviation: GFR, glomerular filtration rate in mL/min/m^2.

Antihypertensive Therapy

ACE inhibitors and angiotensin receptor blockers are considered first-line therapy for hypertension in patients with HIV and chronic kidney disease (12,65) and are safe for use in closely monitored patients with advanced kidney disease (66,67). These agents should be used with caution in the setting of other agents that may promote hyperkalemia, such as pentamidine and trimethoprim, and concomitant use of potassium-sparing diuretics and nonsteroidal anti-inflammatory agents should be avoided.

Expert guidelines recommend the use of two or more antihypertensive agents in most hypertensive patients, particularly those with chronic kidney disease (65). Drug interactions and side-effect profiles should guide the choice of a second antihypertensive agent for older patients with HIV and decreased kidney function. Long-acting or extended release beta blockers may accumulate in patients with reduced GFR and should be avoided in these patients. Calcium channel blockers do not require dose adjustment for GFR, but both diltiazem and verapamil may interfere with the hepatic metabolism of protease inhibitors and other cytochrome P450 CYP3A substrates (68). Diuretics may potentiate both the therapeutic and adverse effects of other antihypertensive agents, and should be used with caution in patients at risk for volume depletion or hyponatremia due to chronic diarrhea or malnutrition. Although loop and thiazide diuretics may be used to manage mild hyperkalemia in patients with chronic kidney disease, potassium-sparing diuretics should generally be avoided in patients with reduced GFR. Alpha blockers do not require dose adjustment for GFR, but anticholinergic effects and orthostatic hypotension limit their tolerability in most patients (65).

Dialysis and Transplantation

Patients with HIV and kidney disease should be referred to a nephrologist with experience in treating this unique patient population. Early referral allows for diagnosis and treatment of specific kidney diseases, as well as general management of chronic kidney disease and its complications. In addition, timely referral facilitates preparation for end-stage renal disease in patients with advanced or progressive kidney disease. The choice of dialysis modality should be based on patient preference, since hemodialysis and peritoneal dialysis offer similar outcomes in patients with HIV and end-stage renal disease (69). With the widespread use of antiretroviral therapy, the one-year survival of HIV-positive dialysis patients is approaching that in the general dialysis population (70). Patients with stage 4 chronic kidney disease (GFR below 30 mL/min/m^2) should select their future dialysis modality to allow time for optimal access placement (58). The preferred hemodialysis access, an arteriovenous fistula, typically requires at least two months for maturation following creation by a vascular surgeon, while training for peritoneal dialysis may require one to two months.

Kidney transplantation is known to confer a significant survival advantage over dialysis in the general end-stage renal disease population. Although it is not yet known whether HIV-infected patients enjoy the same survival advantage, patients with well-controlled HIV and end-stage renal disease should be considered potential candidates for kidney transplantation (71,72), ideally in the context of a clinical trial. Older age is not an absolute contraindication to kidney transplantation, even in the setting of HIV, but suitable candidates should be referred as early as possible because of long waiting times in regions where HIV is prevalent.

Potential kidney transplant candidates with HIV should be on a stable antiretroviral regimen with undetectable HIV viral load, preserved CD4 cell count, and no recent opportunistic infection. Treatment of hepatitis coinfections should be discussed prior to transplantation because of the risk of accelerated cirrhosis with immunosuppressive therapy. Hepatitis C is particularly difficult to treat in the posttransplant setting because of an unacceptably high rate of acute rejection associated with interferon therapy. Following transplantation, close communication between HIV providers and the transplant team is essential to avoid significant drug interactions between immunosuppressive therapy and antiretroviral agents, in particular protease inhibitors and non-nucleoside reverse transcriptase inhibitors (73).

CONCLUSIONS

Kidney disease remains an important complication in the era of antiretroviral therapy and is likely to become increasingly prevalent in our aging patient population. Recognition of kidney disease and communication between HIV providers and nephrologists is essential to avoid complications of kidney disease, to properly adjust medication regimens, and to prepare patients with progressive kidney disease for dialysis or transplantation.

REFERENCES

1. Rao TK, Filippone EJ, Nicastri AD, et al. Associated focal and segmental glomerulosclerosis in the acquired immunodeficiency syndrome. N Engl J Med 1984; 310:669–673.
2. Silva FG. The aging kidney: a review—part I. Int Urol Nephrol 2005; 37:185–205.
3. Silva FG. The aging kidney: a review—part II. Int Urol Nephrol 2005; 37:419–432.
4. Schwartz EJ, Szczech LA, Ross MJ, et al. HAART and the epidemic of HIV+ end stage renal disease. J Am Soc Nephrol 2005; 16:2412–2420.
5. Rowe JW, Andres R, Tobin JD, et al. The effect of age on creatinine clearance in men: a cross-sectional and longitudinal study. J Gerontol 1976; 31:155–163.
6. Franceschini N, Napravnik S, Eron JJ, et al. Incidence and etiology of acute renal failure among ambulatory HIV-infected patients. Kidney Int 2005; 67:1526–1531.
7. Wyatt CM, Arons RR, Klotman PK, et al. Acute renal failure in hospitalized patients with HIV: risk factors and impact on in-hospital mortality. AIDS 2006; 20: 561–565.
8. Wyatt CM, Klotman PE. Antiretroviral therapy and the kidney: balancing benefit and risk in patients with human immunodeficiency virus infection. Expert Opin Drug Saf 2006; 5:275–287.
9. Kopp JB, Miller KD, Mican JA, et al. Crystalluria and urinary tract abnormalities associated with indinavir. Ann Intern Med 1997; 127:119–125.
10. Dieleman JP, Sturkenboom MC, Jambroes M, et al. Risk factors for urological symptoms in a cohort of users of the HIV protease inhibitor indinavir sulfate: the ATHENA cohort. Arch Intern Med 2002; 162(13):1493–1501.
11. Berns JS, Cohen RM, Silverman M, et al. Acute renal failure due to indinavir crystalluria and nephrolithiasis: report of two cases. Am J Kidney Dis 1997; 30: 558–560.
12. Gupta SK, Eustace JA, Winston JA, et al. Guidelines for the management of chronic kidney disease in HIV-infected patients. Recommendations of the HIV Medicine Association of the Infectious Diseases Society of America. Clin Infectious Dis 2005; 40:1559–1585.

13. Chan-Tack KM, Truffa MM, Struble KA, et al. Atazanavir-associated neph-rolithiasis: cases from the US Food and Drug Administration's Adverse Event Reporting System. AIDS 2007; 21(9):1215–1218.
14. Green ST, McKendrick MW, Schmid ML, et al. Renal calculi developing de novo in a patient taking saquinavir. Int J STD AIDS 1998; 9:555.
15. Engeler DS, John H, Rentsch KM, et al. Nelfinavir urinary stones. J Urol 2002; 167:1384–1385.
16. Chugh S, Bird R, Alexander EA. Ritonavir and renal failure. N Engl J Med 1997; 336:138.
17. Duong M, Sgro C, Grappin M, et al. Renal failure after treatment with ritonavir. Lancet 1996; 348:693.
18. Rollot F, Nazal E, Chauvelot-Moachon L, et al. Tenofovir-related Fanconi syndrome with nephrogenic diabetes insipidus in a patient with acquired immunodeficiency syndrome:the role of lopinavir-ritonavir-didanosine. Clin Infect Dis 2003; 37: E174–E176.
19. Ray AS, Cihlar T, Robinson KL, et al. Mechanism of active renal tubular efflux of tenofovir. Antimicrob Agents Chemother 2006; 50(10):3297–3304.
20. Cote HCF, Brumme ZL, Craib KJP, et al. Changes in mitochondrial DNA as a marker of nucleoside toxicity in HIV-infected patients. N Eng J Med 2002; 346:811–820.
21. Morris AA, Baudouin SV, Snow MH. Renal tubular acidosis and hypophosphatemia after treatment with nucleoside reverse transcriptase inhibitors. AIDS 2001; 15:140–141.
22. Saumoy M, Vidal F, Peraire J, et al. Proximal tubular kidney damage and tenofovir: a role for mitochondrial toxicity? AIDS 2004; 18:1741–1742.
23. Vittecoq D, Dumitrescu L, Beaufils H, et al. Fanconi syndrome associated with cidofovir therapy. Antimicrob Agents Chemother 1997; 41:1846.
24. Kahn J, Lagakos S, Wulfsohn M, et al. Efficacy and safety of adefovir dipivoxil with antiretroviral therapy: a randomized controlled trial. JAMA 1999; 282:2305–2312.
25. Gallant JE, Staszewski S, Pozniak AL, et al. Efficacy and safety of tenofovir DF vs stavudine in combination therapy in antiretroviral-naive patients: a 3-year random-ized trial. JAMA 2004; 292:191–201
26. Squires K, Pozniak AL, Pierone G Jr., et al. Tenofovir disoproxil fumarate in nucleoside-resistant HIV-1 infection: a randomized trial. Ann Intern Med 2003; 139:313–320
27. Schooley RT, Ruane P, Myers RA, et al. Tenofovir DF in antiretroviral-experienced patients: results from a 48-week, randomized, double-blind study. AIDS 2002; 16: 1257–1263.
28. Verhelst D, Monge M, Meynard JL, et al. Fanconi syndrome and renal failure induced by tenofovir: a first case report. Am J Kidney Dis 2002; 40:1331–1333.
29. Rifkin BS, Perazella MA. Tenofovir-associated nephrotoxicity: Fanconi syndrome and renal failure. Am J Med 2004; 117:282–284.
30. Barrios A, Garcia-Benayas T, Gonzalez-Lahoz J, et al. Tenofovir-related neph-rotoxicity in HIV-infected patients. AIDS 2004; 18:960–963.
31. Nelson MR, Katlama C, Montaner JSG, et al., for the Tenofovir DF Expanded Access Team. The safety of tenofovir DF for the treatment of HIV infection in adults: the first 4 years. AIDS 2007, 21:1273–1281.
32. Gallant JE, Parish MA, Kennedy JC, et al. Changes in renal function associated with tenofovir disoproxil fumarate treatment, compared with nucleoside reverse-transcriptase inhibitor treatment. Clin Infect Dis 2005; 40:1194–1198.

33. Knudtson E, Para M, Boswell H, et al. Drug rash with eosinophilia and systemic symptoms syndrome and renal toxicity with a nevirapine-containing regimen in a pregnant patient with human immunodeficiency virus. Obstet Gynecol 2003; 101: 1094–1097.
34. Angel-Moreno-Maroto A, Suarez-Castellano L, Hernandez-Cabrera M, et al. Severe efavirenz-induced hypersensitivity syndrome (not-DRESS) with acute renal failure. J Infect 2006; 52:E39–E40.
35. Lalezari JP, Henry K, O'Hearn M, et al. Enfuvirtide, an HIV-1 fusion inhibitor, for drug-resistant HIV infection in North and South America. N Engl J Med 2003; 348:2175–2185.
36. Navarro JF, Quereda C, Quereda C, et al. Nephrogenic diabetes insipidus and renal tubular acidosis secondary to foscarnet therapy. Am J Kidney Dis 1996; 27(3):431–434
37. Farese RV Jr., Schambelan M, Hollander H, et al. Nephrogenic diabetes insipidus associated with foscarnet treatment of cytomegalovirus retinitis. Ann Intern Med 1990; 112:955–956.
38. Schmidt GM, Horak DA, Niland JC, et al. A randomized, controlled trial of pro-phylactic ganciclovir for cytomegalovirus pulmonary infection in recipients of allogeneic bone marrow transplants; The City of Hope-Stanford-Syntex CMV Study Group. N Eng J Med 1991; 324:1005–1001.
39. Sawyer MH, Webb DE, Balow JE, et al. Acyclovir-induced renal failure: clinical course and histology. Am J Med 1988; 84:1067–1071
40. Giustina A, Romanelli G, Cimino A, et al. Low dose acyclovir and acute renal failure. Ann Intern Med 1988; 108:312.
41. Molina JM, Belenfant X, Doco-Lecompte T. Sulfadiazine-induced crystalluria in AIDS patients with toxoplasma encephalitis. AIDS 1991; 5:587–589.
42. Maki DG, Fox BC, Kuntz J, et al. A prospective, randomized, double-blind study of trimethoprim-sulfamethoxazole for prophylaxis of infection in renal transplantation. Side effects of trimethoprim-sulfamethoxazole, interaction with cyclosporine. J Lab Clin Med 1992; 119:11–24.
43. Velazquez H, Perazella MA, Wright FS, et al. Renal mechanism of trimethoprim-induced hyperkalemia. Ann Intern Med 1993; 119:296–301.
44. Allapan R, Perazella MA, Buller GK. Hyperkalemia in hospitalized patients treated with trimethoprim-sulfamethoxazole. Ann Intern Med 1996; 124:316–20.
45. Sattler FR, Cowan R, Nielsen DM, et al. Trimethoprim-sulfamethoxazole compared with pentamidine for treatment of Pneumocystis carinii pneumonia in the acquired immunodeficiency syndrome: a prospective, noncrossover study. Ann Intern Med 1988; 109(4):280–287.
46. Lachaal M, Venuto RC. Nephrotoxicity and hyperkalemia in patients with acquired immunodeficiency syndrome treated with pentamidine. Am J Med 1989; 87:260–263.
47. Kleyman TR, Roberts C, Ling BN. A mechanism for pentamidine-induced hyperkalemia: inhibition of distal nephron sodium transport. Ann Int Med 1995; 122: 103–106
48. Luber AD, Maa L, Lam M, et al. Risk factors for amphotericin B-induced neph-rotoxicity. J Antimicrob Chemother 1999; 43:267–271.
49. Bates DW, Su L, Yu DT, et al. Correlates of acute renal failure in patients receiving parenteral amphotericin B. Kidney Int 2001; 60:1452–9.
50. Linton AL, Clark WF, Driedger AA, et al. Acute interstitial nephritis due to drugs: review of the literature with a report of nine cases. Ann Intern Med 1980; 93:735–741.

51. Mocroft A, Kirk O, Gatell J, et al., for the EuroSIDA study group. Chronic renal failure among HIV-1-infected patients. AIDS 2007; 21:1119–1127.
52. Wyatt CM, Winston JA, Malvestutto C, et al. Chronic kidney disease in HIV infection: an urban epidemic. AIDS 2007; 21:2101–2103.
53. Bruggeman LA, Dikman S, Meng C, et al. Nephropathy in human immunodeficiency virus-1 transgenic mice is due to renal transgene expression. J Clin Invest 1997; 100:84–92.
54. Lucas GM, Eustace JA, Sozio S, et al. Highly active antiretroviral therapy and the incidence of HIV-1-associated nephropathy: a 12-year cohort study. AIDS 2004; 18:541–546.
55. Kimmel PL, Phillips TM, Ferreira-Centeno A, et al. Brief report: idiotypic IgA nephropathy in patients with human immunodeficiency virus infection. N Engl J Med 2002; 327:7026.
56. Haas M, Kaul S, Eustace JA. HIV-associated immune complex glomerulonephritis with "lupus-like" features: a clinicopathologic study of 14 cases. Kidney Int 2005; 67(4):1381–1390.
57. Gerntholtz TE, Goetsch SJW, Katz I. HIV-related nephropathy: a South African perspective. Kidney Int 2006; 69:1885–1891.
58. National Kidney Foundation. K/DOQI clinical practice guidelines for chronic kidney disease: evaluation, classification, and stratification. Am J Kidney Dis 2002; 39:S1.
59. Cockcroft DW, Gault MH. Prediction of creatinine clearance from serum creatinine. Nephron 1976; 16:31–41.
60. Levey AS, Bosch JP, Lewis JB et al. A more accurate method to estimate glomerular filtration rate from serum creatinine: a new prediction equation. Modification of Diet in Renal Disease Study Group. Ann Intern Med 1999; 130:461–470.
61. Bostom AG, Kronenberg F, Ritz E. Predictive performance of renal function equations for patients with chronic kidney disease and normal serum creatinine levels. J Am Soc Nephrol 2002; 13:2140–2144.
62. Wyatt C, Konduri V, Eng J, et al. Reporting of estimated GFR in the primary care clinic. Am J Kidney Dis 2007; 49:634–641.
63. Brown TT, Qaqish RB. Antiretroviral therapy and the prevalence of osteopenia and osteoporosis: a meta-analytic review. AIDS 2006; 20:2165–2174.
64. Leen C, Wat C, Nieforth K. Pharmacokinetics of enfuvirtide in a patient with impaired renal function. Clin Infect Dis 2004; 39:e119–e121.
65. Chobanian, AV, Bakris GL, Black HR, et al. Seventh Report of the Joint National Committee on Prevention, Detection, Evaluation, and Treatment of High Blood Pressure. Hypertension 2002; 42:1206–1252.
66. The GISEN Group (Gruppo Italiano di Studi Epidemiologici in Nefrologia). Randomised placebo-controlled trial of effect of ramipril on decline in glomerular filtration rate and risk of terminal renal failure in proteinuric, non-diabetic nephropathy. Lancet 1997; 349:857–1863.
67. Brenner BM, Cooper ME, de Zeeuw D, et al. Effects of losartan on renal and cardiovascular outcomes in patients with type 2 diabetes and nephropathy. N Engl J Med 2001; 345:861–869.
68. Abernethy DR, Schwartz JB. Calcium-antagonist drugs. N Engl J Med 1999; 341(19):1447–1457.

69. Ahuja TS, Collinge N, Grady J, et al. Is dialysis modality a factor in survival of patients with ESRD and HIV-associated nephropathy? Am J Kidney Dis 2003; 41:1060–1064.
70. Ahuja TS, Grady J, Khan S. Changing trends in the survival of dialysis patients with human immunodeficiency virus in the United States. Am J Kidney Dis 2002; 13:1889–1893.
71. Stock PG, Roland ME, Carlson L, et al. Kidney and liver transplantation in human immunodeficiency virus-infected patients: a pilot safety and efficacy study. Transplantation 2002; 76:370–375.
72. Kumar MSA, Sierka DR, Damask AM, et al. Safety and success of kidney transplantation and concomitant immunosuppression in HIV-positive patients. Transplantation 2005; 67:1622–1629.
73. Jain AK, Venkataramanan R, Shapiro R, et al. The interaction between antiretroviral agents and tacrolimus in liver and kidney transplant patients. Liver Transpl 2002; 8:841–845.

7

The Pulmonary System

Steven Kadiev and Philip T. Diaz
*Division of Pulmonary, Allergy, Critical Care and Sleep Medicine,
Ohio State University, Columbus, Ohio, U.S.A.*

INTRODUCTION

Pulmonary complications are an important source of morbidity and mortality among HIV-infected individuals. While *Pneumocysitis jiroveci* pneumonia represented the most important pulmonary complication through the mid-1990s, the spectrum of pulmonary complications associated with HIV has changed with the advent of highly active antiretroviral therapy (HAART) and improved therapy for HIV (1). With the aging of the HIV population, the spectrum of pulmonary diseases causing important morbidity and mortality continues to evolve. Lung diseases associated with aging, such as chronic obstructive pulmonary disease (COPD) and bronchogenic cancer, appear to be more common in the HIV-seropositive population and will likely become more prevalent as this population ages, particularly given the high prevalence of cigarette smoking among HIV-infected individuals.

This chapter includes a review of changes in pulmonary function and the lung immune environment associated with aging as well as those changes associated with HIV. Specific pulmonary diseases that are linked to aging and significant pulmonary problems for the aging HIV population—COPD, lung cancer, bacterial pneumonia, and *Mycobacterium* tuberculosis (MTB)—are also discussed.

LUNG STRUCTURE AND FUNCTION

Aging-Related Changes

Lung function gradually declines after age 20. There is an increase in the size of the alveolar units and a decrease in the number of capillaries per unit. There is also a decrease in the number of parenchymal elastic fibers, which causes gradual loss of lung elastic recoil. The net result is an increase in both the residual volume and functional residual capacity, while the total lung capacity remains fairly constant (2).

Age-related loss of elastic recoil results in decreased tethering of peripheral airways, which may result in decreased expiratory airflow (3). The gas-exchanging ability of the lungs also deteriorates with age. After early adulthood the carbon monoxide diffusion capacity (DL_{CO}) declines approximately 17% per decade. This reduction is related to the loss of the alveolar-capillary surface area (2). Aging is associated with uniform enlargement of the alveoli with decreased surface area for gas exchange, decreased elastic recoil, and expiratory flow limitation. These changes resemble those seen in emphysema. Nevertheless, in the absence of respiratory insults (such as smoking, exposure to environmental toxins, prior respiratory infections), most elderly people have sufficient respiratory reserve to avoid symptoms (2).

Aging is associated with alterations in the chest wall and respiratory muscles. At about age 55, the chest wall gradually becomes stiffer, resulting in decreased thoracic compliance. This may be due to reduced mobility of the costovertebral joints and intercostal cartilage calcification. There is also development of respiratory muscle weakness related at least in part to decreased intercostal muscle mass (3).

HIV-Related Changes

Investigators studying pulmonary function in the setting of HIV have described pulmonary diffusion impairment (4). Although exacerbated by cigarette smoking, IV drug use, and pneumocystis pneumonia (PCP), an HIV-related drop in diffusing capacity occurs independently of these factors (4,5). Longitudinal studies document that otherwise stable HIV-positive individuals develop large and unexplained "step-like" drops in diffusing capacity for carbon monoxide (DL_{CO}) over a short follow-up period (6). Diaz et al. showed that the DL_{CO} decrement in HIV-positive individuals is consistent with a process that involves destruction of the alveolar capillary interface and correlates with the diffusion impairment of emphysema (7).

Schulz et al. studied respiratory muscle functions, including strength and endurance, in a group of HIV-seropositive individuals (8) and found that HIV-positive subjects had decreased endurance time and lower respiratory muscle strength compared with an age-matched control group. Respiratory muscle weakness was significantly correlated with increased dyspnea (8).

LUNG IMMUNE ENVIRONMENT

The lung is an organ that has constant exposure to the external environment. With a surface area that amounts to approximately 100 m^2, it is necessary to have an efficient and effective immune barrier. Phagocytes, macrophages, and polymorphonuclear neutrophils are major components of inflammatory and immunologic reactions in the lung. Lung macrophages are morphologically and functionally heterogeneous and include alveolar, interstitial, intravascular, and airway macrophages, each with characteristic morphologic and functional features. They play an inflammatory role through the release of cytokines, oxygen radicals, and proteolytic enzymes (9).

Aging-Related Changes

Relatively little is known regarding the local immune changes in the lung that occur with age. Available information suggests that altered immune and inflammatory regulation occurs with aging. Bronchoalveolar lavage studies demonstrate increased total lung lymphocytes and neutrophils and an increase in the CD4/CD8 T-lymphocyte ratio. There is a decrease in B lymphocytes and an increase in immunoglobulin concentrations (3).

Animal and human studies have found alterations in alveolar macrophage function and impaired phagocytosis associated with aging (3). Recent animal data has demonstrated that aging is associated with a delay in the pulmonary cytokine response to respiratory viral infections (10). Aging has also been associated with dysregulation of both pro- and anti-inflammatory cytokine production by alveolar macrophages, as well as an increase in interleukin-6 (IL-6) and in oxidant production by alveolar macrophages. It has been hypothesized that upregulation of macrophage oxidant production may contribute to some observed changes in lung structure and function, including loss of elastic fibers and impairment of gas exchange (3).

HIV-Related Changes

Studies have demonstrated an upregulation of inflammatory events in the lungs of HIV-positive individuals. The occurrence of "lymphocytic alveolitis," characterized by a large increase in BAL CD8$^+$ cytotoxic lymphocytes, has been documented in individuals with HIV (11–14). The increase in CD8$^+$ cells represents a host response to viral antigens with a correlation of the number of CD8$^+$ cells to the viral load in the pulmonary compartment (11). Bronchoalveolar lavage studies have demonstrated that alveolar macrophages are activated in HIV and have an increased capacity to produce cytokines and other inflammatory mediators both spontaneously and in response to a variety of antigenic stimuli (15).

There is an increased inflammatory environment in HIV, but it does not necessarily translate into enhanced immune function. Overall dysfunction of the immune system occurs. Eagan and colleagues have shown that lung fluid immunoglobulin from HIV-infected subjects has impaired ability to "coat" pneumococci, leading to impaired phagocytosis (16). Impaired phagocytosis may explain the increased incidence of invasive pneumococcal pneumonia associated with HIV.

Aging and HIV are associated with alterations in lung function as well as altered immune/inflammatory regulation in the lung. How these changes may affect respiratory physiology in the aging HIV population remains a speculation.

CHRONIC OBSTRUCTIVE PULMONARY DISEASE

The prevalence of COPD in the general population is increasing substantially (17). This is most likely related to past smoking behavior and the aging of the population. The estimated prevalence of cigarette smoking in the HIV-positive population is 50%, over double that in the general population (18). There is evidence that HIV-positive individuals are at increased risk of developing accelerated emphysema (18,19).

Studies support the concept that the alveolar macrophage may play an important role in emphysema pathogenesis (20,21) and that this cell may be central to the pathogenesis of HIV-associated emphysema. In a study of autopsy specimens from patients dying with AIDS, Yearsely et al. found increased numbers of HIV-infected macrophages in areas of pathological emphysema and increased matrix-metalloprotease expression of nearby, noninfected macrophages (22). This suggests that the pathogenesis of HIV-related emphysema may, in part, relate to upregulation of host factors.

Diaz et al. examined high-resolution chest tomography (HRCT) and pulmonary function in 114 HIV-positive subjects and 44 HIV-negative subjects matched for age and smoking history (mean age 34.1 years) (18). There was a high correlation of emphysema to HIV (17/114 compared with 1/44; $P = 0.025$).

Multivariate analysis correlated the risk factors of HIV and pack-year history of cigarette use with the presence of emphysema (18). Thirty-seven percent (14 of 38) of HIV-positive smokers with a history of 12 pack-years or more met the criteria for emphysema, compared with 0% (0 of 14) HIV-negative controls ($P = 0.011$). Forty-six percent (11 of 24) of HIV-positive participants with a smoking history of 25 pack-years or more met the criteria for emphysema, compared with 0% (0 of 10) HIV-negative controls ($P = 0.013$) (Fig. 1).

This prospective study demonstrated the development of an accelerated form of pulmonary emphysema in a stable HIV-positive outpatient sample, and the results suggested that the lesion is related to a heightened susceptibility to cigarette smoke. The concept of a heightened susceptibility to cigarette smoke is corroborated by an analysis of respiratory symptoms among HIV-positive individuals, which documents a marked increase in respiratory symptoms compared with age- and smoking-matched controls (23). It is possible that HIV-associated lung damage involves a similar process as found in non-HIV smokers but that

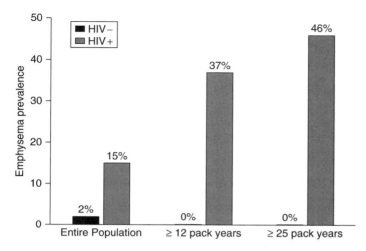

Figure 1 Thirty seven percent (14 of 38) of HIV positive smokers with a smoking history of 12 pack-years or more met criteria for emphysema, compared with 0% (0 of 14) HIV negative controls ($P = 0.011$). Furthermore, 46% (11 of 24) of HIV positive participants with a smoking history of 25 pack-years or more met criteria for emphysema, compared with 0% (0 of 10) in the HIV negative controls ($P = 0.013$).

inflammatory events associated with HIV infection accelerate this process, increasing the likelihood that a smoker with a given pack-year history will develop emphysema.

These observations were made predominantly in the "pre-HAART" era, but data by Crothers et al. (24) have recently confirmed that HIV-positive individuals have a markedly increased risk of COPD in the HAART era. This study of a large cohort of veterans found that HIV infection was associated with a 50% to 60% increased risk of COPD when controlling for confounding variables, including age, smoking, IV drug use, and CD4 count.

Treatment Considerations

There is little information regarding the effects of HAART on immune/inflammatory changes in the lungs of HIV-infected individuals. Since such therapy decreases the lung viral load (25), it is likely to result in a decrease in local lung inflammatory processes with potential implications regarding preservation of lung structure and function.

There are no published studies that have specifically investigated the role of pharmacologic therapy for HIV-associated COPD. However, it is likely that interventions recommended for the general population of COPD patients would be beneficial in patients with HIV. Such a treatment strategy should involve a stepwise approach to symptom management (17). For individuals with minimal symptoms, a short-acting bronchodilator used as needed is reasonable. For those with persistent symptoms despite short-acting agents, long-acting beta-agonists or anticholinergic agents should be used on a regular basis. Patients with persistent symptoms, moderate to severe airflow obstruction, and frequent exacerbations of their COPD may also benefit from inhaled corticosteroids. A multidisciplinary pulmonary rehabilitation program should be employed in subjects with dyspnea despite maximal medical management.

Given the high prevalence of cigarette smoking and the increased susceptibility of HIV-infected individuals to develop parenchymal lung damage, efforts to enhance smoking cessation are imperative. Although there are few studies that have investigated the effectiveness of smoking cessation interventions in the HIV-positive population, available evidence suggests that behavioral and pharmacological interventions can be effective (26,27). Nevertheless, additional investigation and long-term studies are needed to study the effectiveness of various smoking cessation interventions in this special population.

LUNG CANCER

Lung cancer is strongly linked to aging and HIV (28). There are numerous reports demonstrating an increased risk of lung cancer among HIV-seropositive individuals (28–30). The standardized incidence ratio (SIR) for lung cancer among individuals with HIV ranges from 2.0 to 6.5 in most published studies (30).

The etiology of the increased risk has not been elucidated (30). It is difficult to determine if the increased risk is related to the higher prevalence of cigarette smoking in the HIV group, since a number of the existing studies demonstrating the increased risk of lung cancer in the HIV population have not included a suitable control group (29,30). A recent investigation of a large cohort of IV drug abusers suggests that even accounting for smoking history, HIV infection remains an independent risk factor for lung cancer (29).

Kirk et al. reported on the incidence of lung cancer among a large cohort of IV drug abusers in the Baltimore area, followed since 1988 (29). Among over 2086 subjects, 24% were HIV positive and 334 seroconverted over the course of the follow-up period. The investigators identified 27 cases of lung cancer; 14 were in the HIV-seropositive group. After adjusting for smoking and age, the hazard ratio for lung cancer risk among the HIV group was 3.6, suggesting that HIV is an independent risk factor for lung cancer.

Although limited data are available regarding the diagnosis and clinical management of patients with HIV and lung cancer, it appears that HIV patients with lung cancer have a poor prognosis (30). This may be related to diagnosis at an advanced stage, as patients diagnosed with early-stage disease amenable to surgical therapy have outcomes with surgical resection similar to those found in the general non-HIV population (30).

BACTERIAL PNEUMONIA

The majority of excess deaths and hospitalizations due to community-acquired pneumonia (CAP) occur in older adults. The incidence of pneumonia increases dramatically in the very old, from 15 cases per 1000 in those aged 60 to 74 years to 34 cases per 1000 in those 75 years and older (31). Although *Streptococcus pneumoniae, Haemophilus influenzae, Enterobacteriacae*, and *Staphylococcus aureus* are the most frequently identified causative microorganisms, viruses account for up to 26% of hospital admissions for CAP (32). *Chlamydia pneumoniae* has been implicated in CAP and in nursing home–acquired pneumonia (NHAP). Poor oral hygiene increases subsequent risk of pneumonia. Dental plaque may act as a reservoir for pathogenic organisms implicated in CAP or NHAP (32).

Bacterial pneumonia rates are up to 25-fold higher among HIV-infected adults than in the general community, with rates increasing as CD4 cell counts decrease (33). HIV-infected patients with bacteremic pneumococcal pneumonia have a worse 14-day mortality compared with patients who are HIV negative (34). CAP due to *Legionella pneumophilia* has higher morbidity and mortality compared with pneumococcal CAP in HIV-positive patients (35).

While an increase in bacterial pneumonia would be expected to occur in an aging HIV population, the advent of HAART impacts this risk. A retrospective series conducted in France examined the patterns of respiratory disease in HIV individuals in the pre-HAART and HAART eras. Pulmonary opportunistic infections other than PCP and exacerbations of chronic bronchial disease due to gram-negative bacilli virtually disappeared in the HAART era (36). A decline in the incidence of bacterial pneumonia and tuberculosis also occurred (33,37,38).

The pneumococcal polysaccharide vaccine may decrease rates of invasive pneumococcal disease, but this positive effect may be limited to HIV-infected people vaccinated when CD4 cell counts are >500 cells/µL. In sub-Saharan Africa, co-trimoxazole prophylaxis has been shown to reduce the risk of bacterial pneumonia (33).

HIV-induced neutropenia is fairly common, with a wide array of etiologies ranging from infections to toxic chemotherapies. A lower white blood cell count is an independent risk factor for bacterial infection in HIV-positive individuals (39). A randomized, controlled, open-label study using daily filgrastim for HIV-associated neutropenia demonstrated fewer bacterial infections, fewer antibiotic courses, and lower hospital stays and death rates (39).

S. pneumoniae and tuberculosis, two of the most frequent bacterial causes of CAP in the HIV-seropositive population, may have similar clinical presentations. Difficulty in distinguishing the two entities may result in costly and unnecessary empiric antimicrobial therapy. Interestingly, South African data suggests that HIV-positive patients with CAP and a normal procalcitonin level have a low probability of pneumococcal pneumonia, and pulmonary tuberculosis should therefore be actively excluded. The basis of this finding is that pneumococcal CAP invariably has an elevated procalcitonin level, while an elevated level with MTB infection is usually only present if the disease is disseminated (40).

TUBERCULOSIS

The geriatric population represents the largest reservoir of MTB infection in developed nations, including the United States. MTB case rates in the United States are the highest for this age group compared with other age categories. The subtle clinical manifestations of MTB in the elderly can often pose potential diagnostic dilemmas and therapeutic challenges, resulting in increased morbidity and mortality in this age group (41). The institutionalized elderly are at a greater risk, both for reactivation of latent MTB and for the acquisition of new MTB infection. Prevention and control of MTB in facilities providing long-term care to the elderly is therefore imperative (41).

HIV infection is a potent risk factor for MTB. Not only does HIV increase the risk of reactivating latent MTB, it also increases the risk of rapid MTB progression soon after infection (42). HIV-associated MTB also increases MTB transmission rates at the community level. In several countries HIV has been associated with epidemic outbreaks of MTB, and many of the reported outbreaks involved multidrug-resistant strains responding poorly to standard therapy (42). Data suggest that HIV- and MTB-coinfected individuals treated with HAART have comparable survival to non-MTB-infected HIV patients also treated with HAART (43).

Immune reconstitution syndrome (IRS) is especially common in patients with untreated tuberculosis or patients with tuberculosis who have initiated antituberculosis therapy in the past few weeks or months. IRS can be clinically trivial presenting with asymptomatic pulmonary nodules or mediastinal lymph nodes or may be associated with extensive organ dysfunction (1). In one prospective study of HIV-infected patients with active tuberculosis treated with antituberculosis therapy, 36% of the patients treated with HAART versus 7% of the patients not taking HAART developed clinical features consistent with the IRS (1). It appears that the timing of HAART initiation is important with respect to the development of IRS. A recent retrospective analysis concluded that the risk is lower if HAART is initiated after six weeks of antituberculous treatment (7% vs. 54%) (44). Most clinicians would therefore delay the initiation of HAART for four to eight weeks after the start of antituberculosis therapy. Furthermore, the development of IRS is strongly associated with more pronounced HAART-induced CD4 cell count increments and HIV viral load decrements (1). The HIV-positive patients infected with MTB with lower CD4 cell counts should initiate HAART with the caveat that they may develop IRS. However, subjects with higher CD4 cell counts should delay HAART, and those who have cell counts greater than 200 cells/μL should probably defer until antituberculosis therapy is completed (45). IRS has also been reported with the *Mycobacterium avium* complex (1).

CONCLUSIONS

As the HIV-seropositive population ages, the spectrum of HIV-associated pulmonary diseases will evolve. Lung diseases, such as COPD, lung cancer, and community-acquired pneumonia, which are associated with aging and cigarette smoking, may be particularly troublesome in the aging HIV-seropositive population, which has a very high smoking prevalence. In addition, HIV-infected individuals appear to be unusually susceptible to the adverse effects of cigarette smoking. The single most important issue relevant to the natural history of HIV-related pulmonary complications today is the high prevalence of cigarette smoking in this population. Additional research is needed to investigate optimal methods of enhancing smoking cessation in this population.

REFERENCES

1. Grubb JR, Moorman AC, Baker RK, et al. The changing spectrum of pulmonary disease in patients with HIV infection on antiretroviral therapy. AIDS (London, England) 2006; 20:1095.
2. Merck Research Laboratories. The Merck Manual of Geriatrics. Accessed at: http://bibpurl.oclc.org/web/10852http://www.merck.com/pubs/mm%5Fgeriatrics/.
3. Meyer KC. Aging. Proc Am Thoracic Soc 2005; 2:433.
4. Mitchell DM, Fleming J, Pinching AJ, et al. Pulmonary function in human immunodeficiency virus infection. A prospective 18-month study of serial lung function in 474 patients. Am Rev Respir Dis 1992; 146:745.
5. Nieman RB, Fleming J, Coker RJ, et al. Reduced carbon monoxide transfer factor (TLCO) in human immunodeficiency virus type I (HIV-I) infection as a predictor for faster progression to AIDS. Thorax 1993; 48:481–485.
6. Kvale PA, Rosen MJ, Hopewell PC, et al. A decline in the pulmonary diffusing capacity does not indicate opportunistic lung disease in asymptomatic persons infected with the human immunodeficiency virus. Pulmonary Complications of HIV Infection Study Group. Am Rev Respir Dis 1993; 148:390.
7. Diaz PT, King MA, Pacht ER, et al. The pathophysiology of pulmonary diffusion impairment in human immunodeficiency virus infection. Am J Respir Crit Care Med 1999; 160:272–277.
8. Schulz L, Nagaraja HN, Rague N, et al. Respiratory muscle dysfunction associated with human immunodeficiency virus infection. Am J Respir Crit Care Med 1997; 155:1080.
9. Sibille Y, Reynolds HY. Macrophages and polymorphonuclear neutrophils in lung defense and injury. Am Rev Respir Dis 1990; 141:471.
10. Boukhvalova MS, Yim KC, Kuhn KH, et al. Age-related differences in pulmonary cytokine response to respiratory syncytial virus infection: modulation by anti-inflammatory and antiviral treatment. J Infect Dis 2007; 195:511.
11. Twigg HL, Soliman DM, Day RB, et al. Lymphocytic alveolitis, bronchoalveolar lavage viral load, and outcome in human immunodeficiency virus infection. Am J Respir Crit Care Med 1999; 159:1439.
12. Plata F, Autran B, Martins LP, et al. AIDS virus-specific cytotoxic T lymphocytes in lung disorders. Nature (London) 1987; 328:348.

13. Guillon JM, Autran B, Denis M, et al. Human immunodeficiency virus-related lymphocytic alveolitis. Chest 1988; 94:1264.
14. Meignan M, Guillon JM, Denis M, et al. Increased lung epithelial permeability in HIV-infected patients with isolated cytotoxic T-lymphocytic alveolitis. Am Rev Respir Dis 1990; 141:1241.
15. Twigg HL, III. Bronchoalveolar lavage fluid in HIV-infected patients."Cytokine soup." Chest 1993; 104:659.
16. Eagan R, Twigg HL III, French N, et al. Lung fluid immunoglobulin from HIV-infected subjects has impaired opsonic function against pneumococci. Clin Infect Dis 2007; 44:1632.
17. Rabe KF, Hurd S, Anzueto A, et al. Global Strategy for the Diagnosis, Management, and Prevention of Chronic Obstructive Pulmonary Disease: GOLD Executive Summary. Am J Respir Crit Care Med 2007; 176:532–555.
18. Diaz PT, King MA, Pacht ER, et al. Increased susceptibility to pulmonary emphysema among HIV-seropositive smokers. Ann Intern Med 2000; 132:369–372.
19. Diaz PT, Clanton TL, Pacht ER. Emphysema-like pulmonary disease associated with human immunodeficiency virus infection. Ann Intern Med 1992; 116:124.
20. Tetley TD. Macrophages and the pathogenesis of COPD*. Chest 2002; 121: 156S–159S.
21. Russell REK, Culpitt SV, DeMatos C, et al. Release and activity of matrix Metalloproteinase-9 and tissue inhibitor of Metalloproteinase-1 by alveolar macrophages from patients with chronic obstructive pulmonary disease. Am J Respir Cell Mol Biol 2002; 26:602–609.
22. Yearsley MM, Diaz PT, Knoell D, et al. Correlation of HIV-1 detection and histology in AIDS-associated emphysema. Diagn Mol Pathol 2005; 14:48.
23. Diaz PT, Wewers MD, Pacht E, et al. Respiratory symptoms among HIV-seropositive individuals. Chest 2003; 123:1977–1982.
24. Crothers K, Butt AA, Gibert CL, et al. Increased COPD among HIV-positive compared to HIV-negative veterans. Chest 2006; 130:1326–1333.
25. Wood KL, Chaiyarit P, Day RB, et al. Measurements of HIV viral loads from different levels of the respiratory tract. Chest 2003; 124:536.
26. Elzi L, Spoerl D, Voggensperger J, et al. A smoking cessation programme in HIV-infected individuals: a pilot study. Antiviral Ther 2006; 11:787.
27. Wewers ME, Neidig JL, Kihm KE. The feasibility of a nurse-managed, peer-led tobacco cessation intervention among HIV-positive smokers. J Assoc Nurses AIDS Care 2000; 11:37.
28. Engels EA. Human immunodeficiency virus infection, aging, and cancer. J Clin Epidemiol 2001; 54(suppl 1):S29.
29. Kirk GD, Merlo C, O'Driscoll P, et al. HIV infection is associated with an increased risk for lung cancer, independent of smoking. Clin Infect Dis 2007; 45:103.
30. Cadranel J, Garfield D, Lavole A, et al. Lung cancer in HIV infected patients: facts, questions and challenges. Thorax 2006; 61:1000–1008.
31. Krueger P, Loeb M, Kelly C, et al. Assessing, treating and preventing community acquired pneumonia in older adults: findings from a community-wide survey of emergency room and family physicians. BMC Fam Pract 2005; 6:32.
32. Janssens JP. Pneumonia in the elderly (geriatric) population. Curr Opin Pulm Med 2005; 11:226.

33. Feikin DR, Feldman C, Schuchat A, et al. Global strategies to prevent bacterial pneumonia in adults with HIV disease. Lancet Infect Dis 2004; 4:445–455.
34. Feldman C, Klugman KP, Yu VL, et al. Bacteraemic pneumococcal pneumonia: impact of HIV on clinical presentation and outcome. J Infect 2007; 55:125.
35. Pedro-Botet ML, Sopena N, Garcia-Cruz A, et al. Streptococcus pneumoniae and Legionella pneumophila pneumonia in HIV-infected patients. J Infect Dis (Scandinavia)2007; 39:122.
36. Dufour V, Cadranel J, Wislez M, et al. Changes in the pattern of respiratory diseases necessitating hospitalization of HIV-infected patients since the advent of highly active antiretroviral therapy. Lung 2004; 182:331.
37. Wolff AJ, O'Donnell AE. Pulmonary manifestations of HIV infection in the era of highly active antiretroviral therapy. Chest 2001; 120:1888–1893.
38. Mayaud C, Cadranel J. Tuberculosis in AIDS: past or new problems? Thorax 1999; 54:567–571.
39. Kuritzkes DR, Parenti D, Ward DJ, et al. Filgrastim prevents severe neutropenia and reduces infective morbidity in patients with advanced HIV infection: results of a randomized, multicenter, controlled trial. G-CSF 930101 Study Group. AIDS (London, England) 1998; 12:65.
40. Schleicher GK, Herbert V, Brink A, et al. Procalcitonin and C-reactive protein levels in HIV-positive subjects with tuberculosis and pneumonia. Eur Respir J 2005; 25:688–692.
41. Rajagopalan S, Yoshikawa TT. Tuberculosis in long-term-care facilities. Infection Control Hospital Epidemiol 2000; 21:611.
42. Corbett EL, Watt CJ, Walker N, et al. The growing burden of tuberculosis: global trends and interactions with the HIV epidemic. Arch Intern Med 2003; 163:1009–1021.
43. Hung CC, Chen MY, Hsiao CF, et al. Improved outcomes of HIV-1-infected adults with tuberculosis in the era of highly active antiretroviral therapy. AIDS (London, England) 2003; 17:2615.
44. Breen RAM, Smith CJ, Bettinson H, et al. Paradoxical reactions during tuberculosis treatment in patients with and without HIV co-infection. Thorax 2004; 59:704–707.
45. Dean GL, Edwards SG, Ives NJ, et al. Treatment of tuberculosis in HIV-infected persons in the era of highly active antiretroviral therapy. AIDS (London, England) 2002; 16:75.

8

Cancer

David M. Aboulafia

*Virginia Mason Medical Center, University of Washington,
Bailey-Boushay House, Seattle, Washington, U.S.A.*

INTRODUCTION

The risk of certain cancers is increased among those infected with HIV. Four cancers are currently considering AIDS-defining malignancies (ADMs) by the Center for Disease Control (CDC) in Atlanta, Georgia. They are Kaposi's sarcoma (KS), intermediate and high-grade B-cell non-Hodgkin's lymphoma (NHL), primary central nervous system lymphoma (PCNSL), and invasive cervical cancer (1). Each of these malignancies has been associated with infection by viruses other than HIV, including human herpes virus type 8 (HHV-8) in KS (2), Epstein-Barr virus (EBV) in lymphoma (3), and oncogenic types of human papilloma virus (HPV) in cervical cancer (4). Although these viral infections may be necessary for the development of neoplasia, infection alone is not sufficient. Underlying immunosuppression in the host is thought to play an important role in the development of malignancy associated with these organisms (5).

Over the past three decades there has been first a rise and then a fall in the incidence of ADMs in the United States, Europe, and Australia (6–9). The recent decline in ADM incidence as well as other AIDS-defining opportunistic infections has been attributed to the sustained effectiveness of highly active antiretroviral therapy (HAART) (10–12). The effect of potent antiretroviral therapy on the full spectrum of HIV-related cancers continues to be defined (13). If treatment of HIV succeeds in immune restoration, the incidence of some cancers may decline or at least be delayed. However, the reduced morbidity due to HIV infection and longer life expectancy associated with HAART may provide the longer latency period necessary for the development of certain cancers. Several recent studies have demonstrated that non-ADMs account for an increasing proportion of cancer diagnoses in HIV-infected patients, with a proportion of individuals dying as a result of these malignancies increasing from less than 1% in the pre-HAART era to 13% currently (14–17).

The incidence of many common cancers—for example, cancers of the lung, colon, breast, prostate, stomach, and bladder—increases with age in the general population. For 2005, the American Cancer Society (ACS) estimated that the number of new cancer cases in the United States would include 234,460 prostate cancers, 214,640 breast cancers, 174,470 lung cancers, 148,610 colorectal cancers, 58,870 NHLs, and a host of less frequent cancer categories (18). Cancer causes 30% of all deaths in the United States, with the highest mortality rates for lung cancer and several less prevalent cancers such as pancreatic cancer (Fig. 1). Currently 1500 Americans die from cancer complications each day.

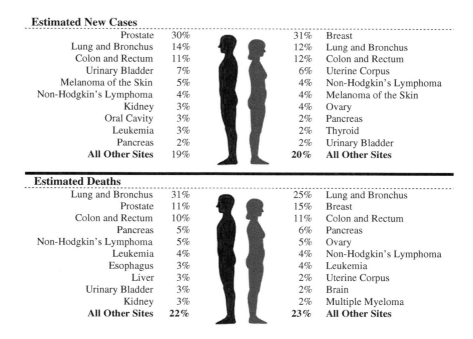

Estimated New Cases

Prostate	30%		31%	Breast
Lung and Bronchus	14%		12%	Lung and Bronchus
Colon and Rectum	11%		12%	Colon and Rectum
Urinary Bladder	7%		6%	Uterine Corpus
Melanoma of the Skin	5%		4%	Non-Hodgkin's Lymphoma
Non-Hodgkin's Lymphoma	4%		4%	Melanoma of the Skin
Kidney	3%		4%	Ovary
Oral Cavity	3%		2%	Pancreas
Leukemia	3%		2%	Thyroid
Pancreas	2%		2%	Urinary Bladder
All Other Sites	19%		**20%**	**All Other Sites**

Estimated Deaths

Lung and Bronchus	31%		25%	Lung and Bronchus
Prostate	11%		15%	Breast
Colon and Rectum	10%		11%	Colon and Rectum
Pancreas	5%		6%	Pancreas
Non-Hodgkin's Lymphoma	5%		5%	Ovary
Leukemia	4%		4%	Non-Hodgkin's Lymphoma
Esophagus	3%		4%	Leukemia
Liver	3%		2%	Uterine Corpus
Urinary Bladder	3%		2%	Brain
Kidney	3%		2%	Multiple Myeloma
All Other Sites	22%		**23%**	**All Other Sites**

Figure 1 Picture summarizing cancer incidence and cancer mortality.

As we enter the third decade of the HIV epidemic and look back on the past 10 years' experience with HAART, it is apparent that several non-ADMs are also linked to HIV infection. Some of the increased incidence may be due to cofactors such as sexually acquired viruses or smoking rather than HIV infection or immunodeficiency per se (9,13,19). Interestingly, of the six mentioned cancers associated with aging, only lung cancer is unequivocally increased in HIV infection arguing against the notion that immunity is important in protecting against all types of cancer.

How best to generalize cancer screening recommendations for the general population to our HIV-infected patients is a moving target. In this chapter, I will very briefly review notions behind cancer pathogenesis as they apply to HIV infection. Recent and important epidemiological studies that provide insight into emerging cancer trends will also be highlighted. This will be followed by specific recommendations for cancer screening as they relate to our aging pool of HIV-infected patients.

PATHOGENESIS

In 1954, Armitage and Dow proposed the multistage model of cancer etiology (20). They maintained that specific changes to a cell's genetic information ("hits") can occur in several ways. These changes may rarely be caused by inborn genetic mutations; more commonly, they are induced by the damaging effects of specific environmental exposures such as cigarette smoke and radiation. Viruses as a type of environmental exposure can supply hits in a unique manner by inserting their own genetic material into a vulnerable cell (21).

Although it is unlikely that HIV acts directly as an oncogenic agent, it may contribute to the development of malignancies through several mechanisms. Impaired immune surveillance, dysregulation of cytokine pathways and growth factor production, chronic B-cell stimulation, and balance between cellular proliferation and differentiation may all contribute to the development of ADMs and AIDS-associated malignancies (22).

In addition, many HIV-associated malignancies affect sites that are in contact with the outside environment (e.g., cervix, lung, oral cavity, skin, anus). The increased density of immune cells in conjunction with elevated concentrations of HIV at these sites could lead to local compromised immune defenses and the subsequent development of malignancies at these sites.

Infection by oncogenic viruses [e.g., cytomegalovirus, EBV, hepatitis B virus (HBV), hepatitis C virus (HCV), and HPV] is also an important risk factor for cancer. For example, not only is HPV an important etiologic factor for anogenital precursor lesions and neoplasia, but recently high-risk HPV infection has been noted in precancerous lesions and squamous cell carcinoma of the conjunctiva in African HIV-positive patients (23). HPV increases the sensitivity of conjunctival cells to ultraviolet-induced mutagenesis (24). HBV DNA can integrate into hepatocyte chromosomal material, which might thereby lead to hepatocellular carcinoma by disrupting key human genes (25). Oncogenic viruses may also act indirectly by interfering with normal cellular processes and by promoting cellular genetic error. For instance, HCV probably increases risk for hepatocellular carcinoma by inducing chronic hepatocellular damage and regeneration, which can then lead to a mutation in a human gene. HIV and HBV/ HCV coinfection is associated with higher serum hepatitis viral RNA levels, faster progression to cirrhosis, and an increased occurrence of hepatocellular carcinoma (26).

The role of immunosuppression in the pathogenesis of NADMs is controversial, particularly as the increased risk of NADMs has been shown in several studies not to be associated with low CD4+ T lymphocyte counts or the onset of AIDS. The potential mutagenic properties of medications (e.g., growth hormone), including HAART, used in the setting of HIV must be considered. As yet there are no data in humans to directly implicate Food and Drug Administration–approved HIV antiretroviral drugs in causing cancer (27). Whether more novel antiretroviral agents such as the chemokine receptor inhibitors (CCR5) are associated with a greater risk of hematologic malignancy is unclear and will require further and careful investigation (28).

Predictors of NADMs appear to be a longer duration of HIV infection, a history of opportunistic infection, and age greater than 40 years. The increased risk with age for many malignancies has a simple explanation under the multistage model of cancer etiology: the age-specific rates of necessary exposures affect the age-specific rates of cancer (20). In the case of cervical cancer, the risk becomes appreciable only after adolescence, the period during which HPV is acquired sexually. Furthermore, although some exposures such as HPV infection are common, the genetic hits that they induce and that are needed for cancer development may be rare and, to some extent, randomly determined (21). Hits might occur only after intense or protracted exposure. Because malignancies occur only with the acquisition of successive hits, cancer incidence increases only after a prolonged period (i.e., with aging). Aging also impairs immune function, albeit to a much smaller degree than does HIV infection, and is associated with increased risk of KS and NHL among HIV-uninfected persons.

Increased risk factors present in the HIV-infected community, including multiple sexual partners, HBV and HCV coinfection, illicit drug use, increased alcohol consumption, and cigarette smoking, could also account for the increased rates of various NADMs (29–31). The effects of cigarette smoking, in particular, must not be underestimated. HIV-positive patients who die of solid tumors are most likely to have smoked. In the Swiss HIV Cohort Study (SHCS), no lung cancers were observed in HIV-positive persons who were nonsmokers (9). Clearly, compared with HIV-infected patients with cancer, more infected patients with cancer have a history of cigarette smoking and recreational drug use.

EPIDEMIOLOGY

Record linkage studies of population-based registries of people with AIDS and cancer have estimated excess cancers for people with AIDS compared with that of the general population. These studies have consistently reported elevated risk for cancers related to oncogenic viruses, including the ADMs, KS, NHL, PCNSL, and, to a lesser extent, invasive cervical cancer, squamous cell cancer of the anus (SCCA), Hodgkin's lymphoma, and liver cancer.

The SHCS, which began collecting data on persons infected with HIV in 1985, observed statistically significant standardized incidence ratios (SIRs) for SCCA (SIR = 33.4), Hodgkin's lymphoma (SIR = 17.3), hepatocellular carcinoma (SIR = 7.0), cancers of the lip, mouth, pharynx, and lung (SIR = 4.1), and non-melanoma skin cancers (SIR = 3.2) (9). In persons infected with HIV, HAART use appeared to minimize the excess risk of KS and NHL, but not that of cervical cancer, Hodgkin's lymphoma, and other NADMs. Among HAART users, the SIR for Hodgkin's lymphoma was comparable to that of KS and NHL. Importantly, cancers of the lung, lip, mouth, or pharynx were not observed among nonsmokers. Data from the California Cancer Registry also showed that compared with the general population, significantly increased cancer incidence rates were observed for SCCA (SIR = 13.4), Hodgkin's lymphoma (SIR = 11.5), liver cancer (SIR = 3.6), oral and respiratory cancers (SIR = 2.6), leukemia (SIR = 2.4), and skin melanomas (SIR = 2.4) (7). As was true in the SHCS, HAART use did not substantially reduce non-ADM risk overall.

Cancer risks in elderly persons with AIDS have not been extensively studied because relatively few elderly persons have developed AIDS. However, in the elderly, cancer incidences rise rapidly and the distribution of cancer types changes with age. Biggar and colleagues investigated cancer risks in persons at least 60 years old at the time of AIDS diagnosis (15). They defined a group as elderly persons with AIDS (EPWAs) to determine whether HIV/AIDS-related immunosuppression affects the profile of cancer risk in the elderly. Compared with the general population, the relative risk (RR) for KS was 545 in the two years after AIDS onset. For NHL, the RR was 24.6. No cervical cancers were reported in this interval. From 60 months before to 27 months after AIDS onset, the RR of non-ADMs was 1.3. The cancer types occurring in significant excess during this period was similar to those of younger adults with AIDS, Hodgkin's lymphoma (RR = 13.1), SCCA (8.2), liver cancer (3.9), multiple myeloma (2.7), leukemia (2.4), and lung cancer (1.9). However, none were significantly elevated in the two years after AIDS onset. Prostate cancer risk was low overall (RR = 0.8). The authors speculated that prostate cancer risk was significantly lower than expected because of reduced screening and follow-up care in EPWAs.

To determine the risk of cancer among HIV-infected women and at-risk HIV-uninfected women, cancer incidence data from the Women's Interagency HIV Study (WIHS) were compared with data from the population-based United States Surveillance, Epidemiology, and End Results (SEER) registry (19).

Among 1554 HIV-infected women, increased incidence rates were observed for KS (SIR = 213.5), NHL (SIR = 19.0), and lung cancer (SIR = 6.3) when compared with SEER rates. The authors recommended that the higher rates of cancer among HIV-infected women, coupled with increased life expectancy, should lead to more intensive cancer screening and prevention efforts in this population. An excess risk was not seen, however, for breast, cervical, and anal cancer in the WIHS.

Population-based registry data have also been used to examine HIV-associated cancer incidence. Among 375,000 people with AIDS in the United States, temporal changes in cancer incidence between 1980 and 2002 were evaluated with researchers specifically focusing on changes occurring in the HAART era (32). Among non-ADMs, lung cancer, Hodgkin's lymphoma, and cancer of the kidney and renal pelvis were most common, with lung cancer representing 24.2% of all cases. Previous studies had also pointed to an elevated risk of lung cancer in HIV infection, with inconclusive results regarding possible changes over time or relationship to HAART use (8,33). A high prevalence of smoking accounts for much of the elevated risk (60–80% of HIV-infected individuals in the United States are smokers), but other factors, including chronic inflammation associated with recurrent infections, may also contribute to the heightened lung cancer risk (34,35).

Unfortunately, important gaps persist in our understanding of cancer risk in HIV-infected individuals. Most linkage studies lack individual data on confounding behavioral risk factors, on biologic markers of immune status and on the use of HAART (9). Uncertainty also arises from the possible biases produced when data are extrapolated from AIDS registries to estimate the risk for all persons infected with HIV, some of whom may never develop AIDS before cancer or death. In contrast, most clinical cohort studies of persons infected with HIV provide detailed individual information on behavioral risk factors, biologic markers, and treatment (36). However, cohort studies often lack the power to detect less frequent cancers and also include selected groups of persons infected with HIV [e.g., women from socioeconomically disadvantaged backgrounds, men who have sex with men (MSM), and hemophiliac men] (9,37,38).

Although studies continue to document dramatic declines in the occurrence of KS and NHL among HIV-infected persons and have attributed these declines to HAART, detailed data on long-term cancer incidence will require further analysis. HIV-infected persons including those who have developed AIDS clearly have an elevated risk for some NADMs such as cancers of the lung, liver, and anus and Hodgkin's lymphoma. While these NADMs are an important source of morbidity, they have been too uncommon for small studies to evaluate thoroughly. Additional data are needed to address the concern that the overall cancer incidence, which generally increases with age, will rise dramatically as people with HIV infection survive longer (32).

While it seems unlikely that the individual components of effective HAART have a differential effect on cancer development, a recent study suggested that how HAART is maintained may impact cancer rates. Among 5472 HIV-infect patients who enrolled in the Strategies for Management of Antiretroviral Therapy (SMART) Study, investigators noted a higher incidence of ADMs but not NADMs among those who underwent a HAART-associated structured treatment interruption (39). The investigators also recorded a higher number of NADMs ($n = 58$) than ADMs ($n = 18$) among study participants. The most common NADMs were skin ($n = 16$), lung ($n = 8$), and prostate ($n = 6$) cancers.

ISSUES IN CANCER SCREENING

Along with increases in survival, the spectrum of underlying causes of death among persons with AIDS has gradually shifted. Between 1987 and 1999, the proportion of deaths due to non-HIV-related causes increased from 10.6 to 22.9 in two U.S. metropolitan areas (14,16). The most common non-HIV-related causes of death reported in the literature are alcohol and drug dependence, cardiovascular disease, and non-HIV-related cancer (40). How best to monitor our aging HIV-infected patients for development of cancer in a cost-effective and efficient manner has not yet been adequately studied.

Professional societies have generally agreed that certain elements of cancer screening are indicated for healthy people with typical risks (Table 1) (41). These recommendations include colon cancer screening, by one of several methods, beginning at 50 years of age; testing for cervical cancer beginning at age 21 or 3 years after sexual activity (whichever comes sooner); and mammography to detect early breast cancer beginning between the age of 40 and 50 years. Various metrics for prostate cancer screening have also been proposed. At present, the ACS or other medical or scientific organizations do not routinely recommend testing for early lung cancer detection in asymptomatic individuals. Prospective trials to evaluate the efficacy of spiral computed tomography are under way in the United States and Europe, with results expected before the end of the decade (42).

Formal guidelines for screening HIV-infected patients for colon, breast, and prostate cancer have not yet been formulated. For HIV-infected women, various groups, including the ACS and the American College of Obstetricians and Gynecologists (ACOG), have provided cervical cancer screening guidelines (41,43). Most recently, the New York Health Department issued controversial recommendations for anal cancer screening for HIV-infected men and women (44).

Although there are data to show that cancer screening is generally neglected in the setting of HIV infection, data to attest to its benefits are scant. Nonetheless, as we await a clearer understanding of cancer risk and the natural history of various NADMs in those infected with HIV, it is prudent to offer, at the least, similar cancer screening surveillance that we provide average-risk asymptomatic non-HIV-infected patients in the case of breast, colon, and

Table 1   American Cancer Society Recommendations for the Early Detection of Cancer in Average-Risk Asymptomatic People

Cancer site	Population	Test or procedure	Frequency
Breast	Women aged ≥ 20 years	BSE	Beginning in their early 20s, women should be told about the benefits and limitations of BSE. The importance of prompt reporting of any new breast symptoms to a health professional should be emphasized. Women who choose to do BSE should receive instruction and have their technique reviewed on the occasion of a periodic health examination. It is acceptable for women to choose not to do BSE or to do BSE irregularly.
		CBE	For women in their 20s and 30s, it is recommended that CBE be part of a periodic health examination, preferably at least every 3 years. Asymptomatic women aged ≥ 40 years should continue to receive a clinical breast examination as part of a periodic health examination, preferably annually.
		Mammography	Begin annual mammography at age 40 years[a]
Colorectal	Men and women aged ≥ 50 years	FOBT[b] *or* FIT, *or* flexible sigmoidoscopy, *or* FOBT[b] and flexible sigmoidoscopy,[c] *or* DCBE, *or* colonoscopy	Annual, starting at age 50 years Every 5 years, starting at age 50 years Annual FOBT (or FIT) and flexible sigmoidoscopy every 5 years, starting at age 50 years DCBE every 5 years, starting at age 50 years Colonoscopy every 10 years, starting at age 50 years
Prostate	Men aged ≥ 50 years	DRE and PSA test	The PSA test and the DRE should be offered annually, starting at age 50 years, for men who have a life expectancy of at least 10 years.[d]

Table 1 American Cancer Society Recommendations for the Early Detection of Cancer in Average-Risk Asymptomatic People (*Continued*)

Cancer site	Population	Test or procedure	Frequency
Cervix	Women aged ≥ 18 years	Pap test	Cervical cancer screening should begin approximately 3 years after a woman begins having vaginal intercourse, but no later than age 21 years. Screening should be done every year with conventional Pap tests or every 2 years using liquid-based Pap tests. At or after age 30 years, women who have had three normal test results in a row may get screened every 2 to 3 years with cervical cytology (either conventional or liquid-based Pap test) alone, or every 3 years with a HPV DNA test, plus cervical cytology. Women aged ≥ 70 years who have had three or more normal Pap tests and no abnormal Pap tests in the last 10 years and women who have had a total hysterectomy may choose to stop cervical cancer screening.

[a]Beginning at age 40 years, annual clinical breast examination should be performed prior to mammography.

[b]FOBT, as it is sometimes done in physicians' offices with the single stool sample collected on a fingertip during a DRE, is not an adequate substitute for the recommended at-home procedure of collecting two samples from three consecutive specimens and is not recommended. Toilet bowl FOBT tests also are not recommended. In comparison with guaiac-based tests for the detection of occult blood, immunochemical tests are more patient-friendly and are likely to be equal or better in sensitivity and specificity. There is no justification for repeating FOBT in response to an initial positive finding. Patients with a positive screening FOBT should undergo colonoscopy.

[c]Flexible sigmoidoscopy together with FOBT is preferred compared with FOBT or flexible sigmoidoscopy alone.

[d]Information should be provided to men about the benefits and limitations of testing so that an informed decision about testing can be made with the clinician's assistance.

Abbreviations: BSE, breast self-examination; CBE, clinical breast examination; FOBT, fecal occult blood test; FIT, fecal immunochemical test; DCBE, double-contrast barium enema; DRE, digital rectal examination; PSA, prostate-specific antigen; HPV, human papilloma virus.

prostate cancer, and heightened surveillance in the case of cervical and possibly anal cancer.

CERVICAL CANCER

Cervical cancer is second only to breast cancer in being the most common cancer among women worldwide. Almost 80% of cases occur in developing countries, and in many regions it is the most common cancer among women (45). Cervical cancer is less common in economically developed countries, where screening programs have been in existence for several decades. In the United States, the majority of cervical carcinoma patients are diagnosed with early-stage disease. Among the 13,458 staged patients with cervical cancer registered by SEER between 1973 and 1987, 71% were diagnosed with International Federation of Gynecology and Obstetrics (FIGO) stage I–IIA tumors (46). Most of these women with early lesions are cured with surgery or radiation alone (47).

In addition to annual examinations, the ACS and ACOG recommend annual screening with conventional Papanicolao (Pap) or thin prep tests for cervical cancer for women younger than 30 years (Table 1) (41,43). For those 30 years or older, screening options consist of annual cytology and less frequent screening (every 2–3 years) in those with three consecutive normal test results and who test negative for oncogenic HPV DNA. The recommended interval is 6 to 12 months for women with normal cytology results and detectable oncogenic HPV. If an HPV test is not obtained, three consecutive normal Pap smear results are required before the Pap smear frequency is changed to once every two or three years (48).

While HPV infection is common in the general population, it is even more common among those who are infected with HIV. Among 112 HIV-infected women enrolled in the Study to Understand the Natural History of HIV/AIDS in the Era of Effective Therapy (SUN), 86% had cervical HPV infection (49). Although it is generally considered a sexually transmitted infection, HPV may be spread through nonsexual skin-to-skin contact. Condoms are only partially effective in preventing HPV transmission, since infection can occur through uncovered areas. Infected individuals may transfer the virus even if they have no visible external warts. Infants born to infected mothers may also contract HPV during delivery (50).

In most healthy HIV-negative individuals, the immune system is able to keep HPV infection under control and the infection is asymptomatic (51). But HIV-infected women—particularly those with more advanced disease—have more persistent HPV, are more likely to develop HPV-related dysplasia, have a faster rate of progression to cancer, and are more likely to experience recurrence after treatment (52).

The natural progression of persistent oncogenic HPV DNA on the cervix to cervical intraepithelial neoplasia (CIN) among HIV-infected women is now well established. Several case control studies have demonstrated a 2 to 12 times higher cytological abnormality rate against control HIV-seronegative women (53,54). Furthermore, in a longitudinal study of HIV-infected women, Delmas and colleagues reported the natural history of HPV infection and preinvasive disease of the cervix (55). Women with CD4+ T-lymphocyte counts less than 200 cells/µL had a twofold increase in both prevalence and incidence of CIN compared with women with CD4+ T-lymphocyte counts greater than 500 cells/µL. In a study of 307 HIV-positive women, high HPV viral load was associated with a 10-fold increased risk of CIN among women with severe immunosuppression than among those with higher CD4+ T-lymphocyte cell counts (56).

In examining the cumulative incidence of CIN according to baseline HPV DNA, HIV serostatus, and CD4+ T-lymphocyte cell count, the WIHS showed that among 855 HIV-infected women, the incidence of CIN in those with CD4+ T-lymphocyte counts below 500 cells/µL was greater than in 343 women without HIV infections on multivariate analysis; the rate of CIN in HIV-infected women with higher CD4+ T-lymphocyte cell counts was comparable to that in HIV-seronegative women (57). For those women enrolled in the WIHS with normal Pap tests and undetectable HPV at baseline, 29% of HIV-positive women with CD4+ counts below 200 cells/µL developed CIN over three years compared with 14% of those with 200 to 500 cells/µL, 6% of those with more than 500 cells/µL. In contrast, 5% of HIV-seronegative women with normal Pap tests and undetectable HPV at baseline developed CIN over three years.

The relationship between HIV and cervical cancer is unique in that women at risk for both conditions share common sociobehavioral patterns such as early onset of sexual intercourse, high number of sexual partners, and smoking (58). The persistence of high risk or oncogenic HPV types (types 16, 18, 31, 33, 35, 39, 45, 51, 52, 56, 58, 59, 66, 68) on the cervix results in manipulation of cell cycle control and malignant transformation, now estimated to last up to 15 years when immunosurveillance is normal.

HAART has the potential to prevent progression of HPV infection and subsequent induction of regression of CIN lesions. Yet the precise beneficial effect of HAART on HPV infection and CIN lesions remains uncertain (52). In a study of 168 HIV-positive women, of whom 96 were receiving HAART, there was 40% regression of CIN (59). In another study of 71 HIV-positive women receiving HAART, there was a 13% regression of CIN without treatment of the cervix, and a greater increase in CD4+ cell counts was significantly associated with regression (60). In general, these studies suggest that HAART has a modest impact on HPV-related disease progression. Epidemiologic surveys indicate that the overall incidence of invasive cervical cancers have remained unchanged or tended to increase in the HAART era (61).

Guidelines for cervical cancer screening for HIV-seropositive women have not been revised since 1995. For now and until appropriate clinical trial data are available, the existing recommendations regarding surveillance of lower genital tract neoplasia in HIV-infected women should generally be followed (41,43,44,62,63). These include inspection of the external anogenital area as part of the annual physical exam and taking of biopsies of all suspicious external lesions for histopathologic assessment. For women with newly diagnosed HIV infection, two Pap tests at six-month intervals should be obtained within the first year. If the results of both are negative, cytologic tests can be repeated annually in those women with CD4+ counts greather than 500 cells/µL.

In women with lesser CD4+ cell counts and those with abnormal Pap findings, Pap tests should be done every six months. Colposcopy should be performed in all cases in which Pap testing reveals atypical squamous cells of undetermined significance (ASCUS) or worse. CIN should be treated with excisional techniques (loop electrosurgical excision procedure) being favored over cryosurgery. Localized vulvar and intraepithelial neoplasia should be treated conservatively—for example, with carbon dioxide laser vaporization, fulguration, or trichloroacetic acid. Trichloroacetic acid is non-teratogenic and can be safely used during pregnancy or in women who might become pregnant. Because of a high rate of recurrence after surgery, extensive external anogenital lesions should be monitored biannually (58).

HPV test results have traditionally not been considered in frequency of Pap assessments, even though economic models have suggested that HPV testing in HIV-seropositive women might be cost effective. In the WIHS, a similar low cumulative incidence of any squamous intraepithelial lesion was observed among HIV-seronegative and HIV-seropositive women with CD4+ T-lymphocyte counts greater than 500 cells/µL and who had normal cervical cytology and HPV-negative test results (57). Similar cervical cancer screening practices may be applicable to both groups, but further study of this issue is needed.

ANAL CANCER

Over the past 20 to 30 years, the incidence of SCCA in the United States has increased by 96% in men and 39% in women (64). Prior to the HIV pandemic, among MSM, the incidence of SCCA had been estimated to be 35 cases per 100,000 population, which is comparable to the incidence of cervical cancer before the introduction of routine cervical Pap screening (65). On the basis of studies in both Europe and the United States, the risk for anal cancer among HIV-infected MSM has been estimated to be twice that among non-HIV-infected MSM (66,67). Furthermore, the incidence of anal cancer in HIV-infected MSM appears to be increasing in the HAART era (68).

Anal HPV infection appears to be most common among MSM, but it also occurs in women and men who do not practice anal sex. Kojic and colleagues found that anal HPV infection was more common than cervical infection in HIV-positive women including those who did not have anal sex (49). On the whole, more women than men develop anal cancer each year (63).

HIV and HPV coinfected patients are at high risk of developing pre-cancerous anal lesions (AIN) and invasive anal malignancies. Analogous to HIV-infected women with HPV-associated cervical changes, the longer life expectancy of these coinfected individuals in the era of HAART provides an opportunity for invasive SCCA to develop from its dysplastic precursor. On the basis of multiple epidemiologic and histopathologic associations, SCCA is thought to behave like cervical cancer (52). Both anal and cervical cancer share an etiologic link to high-risk types of HPV infection and share similar cytologic rating systems for dysplasia (69,70).

The prognosis of SCCA, like that of many other cancers, is strongly associated with the stage of disease at diagnosis. A recent analysis of anal cancer outcomes from 1972 through 2000 found that survival was significantly improved for patients who received a diagnosis of local disease (5-year survival rate, 78%) than for those who received a diagnosis of regional disease (5-year survival rate, 56%) or distant disease (5-year survival rate, 18%) (64). Concomitant radiation therapy and chemotherapy is the current standard of care of HIV-negative patients with invasive anal carcinoma, and this approach has been investigated and applied successfully to HIV-positive patients with similar anal cancers, particularly those with CD4+ T-lymphocyte count greater than 200 cells/μL (71,72).

Although low-grade anal dysplasia has been shown to progress to high-grade dysplasia in a majority of HIV-infected men within two years after initial diagnosis, the true rate of progression from high-grade dysplasia to invasive anal cancer remains unclear. Similar to the findings seen in HIV-infected women with HPV-associated cervical dysplasia, studies suggest that HAART has a modest impact on HPV-related anal disease progression. One French study, for example, found that the use of HAART did not lead to the regression of precancerous anal lesions or HPV clearance in HIV-positive men (73). At a minimum, HIV-positive persons, whether or not they are receiving HAART, need to continue to be observed closely because they remain at risk of developing high-grade AIN.

Using the cervical paradigm, screening for anal cytological abnormalities, defining the abnormality pathologically by anal biopsy, and subsequently treating potentially premalignant lesions have been proposed as a management strategy to prevent the progression of high-grade dysplasia to anal cancer. Anal screening has similar sensitivity to cervical cytology screening in HIV-positive MSM to detect the presence of dysplastic cells (74).

With these issues in mind, the New York Health Department recently became the first state health department to recommend anal Pap smear screening as a standard intervention in high-risk groups, including MSM and HIV-positive individuals (44). However, no randomized clinical trials exist to support anal Pap smear screening. A prospective randomized control trial evaluating anal Pap smears would need to be very large and would take many years to complete (70). Nonetheless, as trials that seek to evaluate treatment strategies for high-grade anal dysplasia mature, it is likely that anal Pap assessments will become a standard of care for high-risk groups analogous to cervical Pap assessments for women.

Anal Pap smear screening involves inserting a swab blindly into the anal canal and fixing the cells either on a slide or fluid for liquid cytological examination (75,76). Anal cytology is classified on the basis of the revised Bethesda system of cervical cytology classification: normal, ASCUS, low-grade squamous intraepithelial lesions (SILs), or high-grade SILs.

HIV-positive patients with normal anal Paps are screened yearly. All abnormal anal cytology is referred for high-resolution anoscopy (HRA). In the same manner that patients with cervical cytologic abnormalities undergo colposcopy and direct visualization and biopsy of any suspect lesions, the anus and perianal region is examined with HRA. Berry and colleagues developed this technique at the University of California, San Francisco, beginning in the early 1990s (77). HRA is easily performed in the outpatient setting using a colposcope and requires no preparation by the patient. HRA can be used in the operating room to guide detection and treatment of anal dysplasia using an operating microscope. In the clinic, patients lie in the left lateral decubitus position at the end of the examination table while bracing their feet in one of the stirrups. After obtaining a Pap smear, a digital rectal exam (DRE) is performed using a combination of lubricating jelly and 2% lidocaine jelly to minimize the discomfort associated with the vinegar. A regular disposable plastic anoscope is inserted but then removed after placing a wooden Dacron swab into the anal canal through the anoscope for one minute with a thin piece of gauze wrapped around the end that is saturated with 3% acetic acid. The anoscope is reinserted after removing the gauze swab, and the anal canal is examined carefully using a colposcope with 6×25 magnification. The squamocolumnar junction is easily visualized and carefully inspected because this location is where most high-grade SILs are found. Tissue samples of any suspicious lesions are collected using either endoscopic biopsy forceps or tissular biopsy forceps. Bleeding is usually minimal and controlled by removing the anoscope or by applying Monsel solution, which promotes coagulation.

The aim of anal cytology testing is to detect either normal or abnormal results, as anal cytology grade is poorly predictive of anal dysplasia grade following HRA and biopsy, and should not be relied upon without histological confirmation (75,77).

By routinely performing anal Pap tests and carefully evaluating the anal canal with HRA, we hope that the risk of SCCA will be ameliorated among HIV-infected persons. Low-grade dysplasia on biopsy is followed up at six-month intervals with HRA due to the high rate of progression from low-grade to high-grade dysplasia. High-grade dysplasia on biopsy is treated or followed depending on the size of the lesion (Fig. 2) (78). Not lost in the assessment of cervical and anal cancer dysplasia is the important role that the medical provider must play in seeking to modify cancer-promoting activities in this population (Table 2) (50).

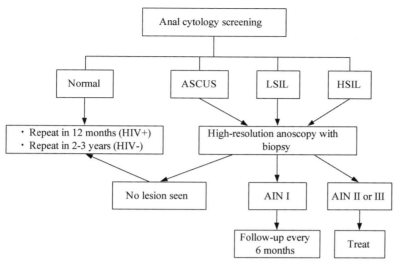

ASCUS = atypical squamous cells of uncertain significance

LSIL = low-grade squamous intraepithelial lesions

HSIL = high-grade squamous intraepithelial lesion

AIN = anal intraepithelial neoplasia

Figure 2 Anal cancer screening algorithm. *Abbreviations*: ASCUS, atypical squamous cells of uncertain significance; LSIL, low-grade squamous intraepithelial lesions; HSIL, high-grade squamous intraepithelial lesion; AIN, anal intraepithelial neoplasia.

Table 2 Cervical and Anal Cancer Prevention Tips

- Smoking is a known risk factor for cervical and anal cancer.
- Having multiple sex partners increases the risk of HPV infection.
- While not completely protective, condoms can lower the risk of HPV infection and reinfection with new types.
- Women with multiple partners should consider a contraceptive method other than the pill, which may increase the risk of HPV infection.
- Women should get regular Pap smears (every 6–12 months if HIV positive; at least every three years if HIV negative).
- At-risk men should get regular anal exams and ask their doctor about anal Pap smears.
- If Pap test results are abnormal, get a follow-up colposcopy or anoscopy.

Abbreviation: HPV, human papilloma virus.

COLORECTAL CANCER

Colorectal cancer (CRC) is the second leading cause of cancer-related death in the United States; each year approximately 150,000 new cases of CRC are diagnosed, and over 50,000 persons die from the disease (77). It is estimated that a person dying of CRC loses 14 years of life.

Current screening guidelines from the U.S. Preventive Services Task Force (80), the ACS (41), and others (81) recommend CRC screening starting at age 50 for all persons at average risk for CRC. There are a number of options for colorectal screening that may be chosen on the basis of individual risk, personal preference, and access (Table 1). For example, the ACS recommends that average-risk adults should begin colorectal screening at age 50 years, with one of the following options: (1) fecal occult blood testing (FOBT) with either guaiac or immunohistochemical-based test following manufacturer's recommendations for specific collection, (2) flexible sigmoidoscopy every 5 years, (3) annual FOBT plus flexible sigmoidoscopy every 5 years, (4) double contrast barium enema every 5 years, or (5) colonoscopy every 10 years (41). Single-panel FOBT in the medical office using a stool sample collected during a digital rectal exam is not a recommended option because of its very low sensitivity for advanced adenomas and cancer.

The ACS and other organizations further recommend more intense surveillance for individuals at higher risk for colorectal cancer (41). Individuals at high risk for colorectal cancer include those (1) with a history of adenoma polyps, (2) with a personal history of cured or resected CRC, (3) with a family history of either CRC or colorectal adenomas diagnosed in a first-degree relative before age 60 years, (4) at significantly high risk due to a history of inflammatory bowel disease of significant duration, or (5) at significantly higher risk due to a known or suspected presence of one of two hereditary syndromes, specifically hereditary nonpolyposis colon cancer or familial adenomatosis polyposis. For these individuals, increased surveillance generally means a specific recommendation for colonoscopy, if available, and may include more frequent exams beginning at an earlier age.

Reported data on the relationship between CRC and HIV-infected patients are emerging. Several studies have suggested that CRC is one of the non-ADMs that may be increasing in the HIV-seropositive population. For example, a prospective study of 2882 patients with HIV found that the annual incidence of CRC was 0.65 per 1,000 patients-years in the pre-HAART era, and this increased to 2.34 per 1,000 patient-years between 1997 and 2002 (82). In contrast, other studies suggest that the incidence of CRC is not higher in HIV-infected patients than in the general population and that, when compared with the pre-HAART era, there been no increase in CRC incidence in HIV-infected patients (8,9,15,32). These contradictory findings highlight the need for large, well-designed studies to evaluate CRC in this population.

Information about the presentation, clinical course, and response to therapy in HIV patients with CRC is also limited. In one case-control study of 3951 CRC patients, 12 HIV seropositive CRC patients (0.3%) were identified (83). The HIV-positive CRC patients tended to be younger, have a more aggressive clinical presentation, and have a less favorable outcome than their HIV-negative counterparts. In another study, the median age at the time of diagnosis of CRC was 51 years in HIV-infected patients compared with 69 years in those without HIV (84). Yeguez and colleagues found that the median age of HIV-infected patients with adenocarcinoma of the colon was even younger (46 years), and four of the six patients were younger than 40 years (85).

Although many HIV-infected patients are living well beyond 50 years of age, there are limited published data on CRC screening in this population (86). Among patients at a Veterans Administration Medical Center, 538 HIV-infected outpatients were seen during an 18-month period (85). Three hundred and two (56%) were older than 50 years. Despite significantly more visits with their primary care provider, HIV-infected patients were less likely than their HIV-negative counterparts to have ever had at least one CRC screening test (56% vs. 78%, $p < 0.001$). The proportion of HIV-infected patients who had ever had a FOBT (43% vs. 67%, $p < 0.001$), flexible sigmoidoscopy (5.3% vs. 17.5%, $p < 0.001$), air contrast barium enema (2.6% vs. 7.9%, $p = 0.004$), or a colonoscopy (17.2% vs. 27.5%, $p = 0.002$) was significantly lower than in control subjects. In addition, HIV-infected patients were significantly less likely to be up to date with at last one CRC screening according to current guidelines (49% vs. 66%, $p < 0.001$). Older age, a family history of CRC, more than 10 visits with their primary care provider in the past 24 months, and an undetectable HIV viral load were the variables that were significantly associated with ever having at least one CRC screening test. These findings are not surprising because older patients and those with a family history of CRC are at increased risk of developing cancer of the colon and rectum and are probably more likely to be offered and to accept screening.

Veterans Administration investigators have also evaluated the prevalence of colonic neoplasms detected by flexible sigmoidoscopy among patients with HIV and determined factors associated with colonic neoplasms in this population. Among 2382 patients, 165 were HIV positive and the prevalence of adenomas in the distal colon was significantly higher in HIV-infected patients than in control subjects (20% vs. 13%, $p < 0.001$), and the odds of HIV-infected patients having a neoplastic lesion (7% vs. 4%, $p = 0.03$) were significantly higher even after adjustment for potential confounding variables (87). Among individuals with positive results on flexible sigmoidoscopy, proximal colonic neoplastic lesions on follow-up colonoscopy were more common in HIV-infected patients after adjustments for age, sex, and race/ethnicity (odds ratio, 1.88).

As life expectancy of persons with HIV continues to increase, a better understanding of etiology, epidemiology, and natural history of colorectal polyps and cancers will be necessary in order to implement age-appropriate CRC prevention, screening, and treatment recommendations. In the meantime, apply colon cancer screening guidelines for HIV-infected patients in a manner and frequency that is customary for non-HIV-infected individuals.

BREAST CANCER

Breast cancer is the most common female cancer in the United States, the second most common cause of cancer death in women, and the main cause of death in women aged 45 to 55 years (88). The most important risk factors are family history and hormonal factors.

A majority of breast cancers are diagnosed as a result of an abnormal mammogram. Further evaluation (accessory mammographic projections, ultrasound, magnetic resonance imaging) may be needed to determine the need for tissue biopsy. The goal of the initial biopsy is to obtain diagnostic material using the least invasive approach and to avoid excising benign lesions. An important point that cannot be overemphasized is that up to 20% of new breast cancers are not detected or visible on mammograms. Therefore, a suspicious lump should not be disregarded just because the mammogram is negative (89).

Breast cancer has been reported in both HIV-positive women and men. Like many other NADMs, the incidence of breast cancer among HIV-infected women is not well defined. Initial case reports involving HIV-positive women with breast cancer described an early age of onset, a propensity for unusual or poorly differentiated neoplasms, early metastases, and poor survival outcome (27). Subsequent studies have suggested a different clinical picture. In a recent series of HIV-infected patients who presented with early breast cancer (stage I and II), the five-year survival rate (80%) was similar to that of an HIV-indeterminate (control) group of patients (90). HIV-infected breast cancer patients should probably be treated in a fashion similar to their non-HIV-infected counterparts, particularly when they have CD4+ counts greater than 200 cells/μL and controlled HIV viral loads (91).

Between the ages of 20 and 39 years, the ACS recommends that women undergo clinical breast examination every 3 years and annually after age 40 years (Table 1) (41). This exam, which should take place during periodic health examinations, provides an opportunity for a health care professional to review and update the family history, discuss the importance of early breast cancer detection, and answer questions women may have about their own risk, new technologies, and other matters related to breast disease. The ACS further advises that during these discussions, health care professionals emphasize the importance of awareness and recognition of breast changes and, if changes occur, to instruct women to contact their medical providers promptly. Although the ACS no longer recommends monthly breast self-examination (BSE), women should be informed about the potential benefits, limitations, and harms (principally, the possibility of false-positive result) associated with BSE. Women may then choose to do BSE regularly, occasionally, or not at all. If a woman chooses to perform periodic BSE, she should receive instructions in the technique and have her technique reviewed periodically (89).

Per the ACS, average-risk women should begin annual mammography at the age of 40 years (Table 1) (41). Women should also be informed about the scientific evidence demonstrating the value of detecting breast cancer before symptoms develop and the importance of adherence to a schedule of regular mammograms. Benefits include a reduction in the risk of dying from breast cancer, less invasive therapy, and a greater range of treatment options. Women also should be told about the limitations of mammography, specifically that mammography will not detect all breast cancers and that some breast cancers detected with mammography may still have poor prognoses. Further, women should be informed about the potential harms associated with mammographic screening, including false positives, biopsy for abnormalities that prove to be benign, and the short period of anxiety that typically will accompany the uncertainty about the presence of malignancy (89).

As with cervical cancer screening guidelines, there is no specific upper age at which mammography screening in HIV-infected women should be discontinued. Rather, the decision to stop regular mammography screening should be individualized on the basis of the potential benefits and risks of screening in the context of overall health status and estimated longevity. As long as a woman is in good health and would be a candidate for breast cancer treatment, she should continue to be screened with mammography.

Available tools like the Gail model of breast cancer risk take into accounts various factors such as the patient's age, race, family history, and findings on previous breast biopsies to provide an estimate of cancer risk (92). The Gail model is readily downloadable from the World Wide Web, and relevant patient variables can be entered into a computer program to provide a 5- and 10-year risk assessment of breast cancer development. Although this model has proven valuable in the assessment of non-HIV-infected women, it has not been validated in the setting of HIV infection.

In a recent comprehensive review of HIV-related breast disease, Gewurz and colleagues emphasized an important issue: because of various reasons including socioeconomic disadvantages in HIV-infected women, these patients often do not receive adequate screening mammography (91). This is borne out by two recent studies. In the first, among women monitored at the Johns Hopkins University Moore Clinic, only 56% of eligible HIV-infected women were referred for screening mammography (93). In the second study, investigators used data from the WIHS to compare 2059 HIV-positive women with 569 HIV-negative women on use of mammography. They also compared mammography used between WIHS women and U.S. women in general using National Health Insurance Survey (NHIS) data (94). Among women aged 40 years or older, fewer WIHS women, regardless of HIV status, reported screening than U.S. women (67% HIV-positive, 62% HIV-negative, 79% NHIS; $p < 0.0001$). The authors concluded: "Breast cancer incidence will almost certainly increase among HIV-positive women as a consequence of improved survival due to efficacious antiretroviral therapy. Primary care physicians and other health care providers, such as nurses and physician assistants, need to be educated about the importance of mammography for HIV-positive women.

Stereotypes die slowly, and many health care providers may not realize how long women are living with HIV-infection."

PROSTATE CANCER

Prostate cancer is the most common malignancy diagnosed in American men and the third leading cause of male cancer mortality. According to the ACS, an estimated 218,890 men will be diagnosed and 27,050 will die from prostate cancer in the United States in 2007 (41). One in six men will be diagnosed with prostate cancer in his lifetime, and one in 34 men will die of prostate cancer.

A substantial number of elderly men are getting screened for prostate cancer unnecessarily. In a cohort study involving nearly 600,000 men aged 70 years and older at dozens of Veterans Administration hospitals in the United States, investigators noted high rates of prostate-specific antigen (PSA) testing, even among elderly men with multiple comorbidities whose life expectancy was substantially less than 10 years (95). Men with a history of prostate cancer, elevated PSA, or symptoms of the disease were excluded from the analysis.

Recently, the ACS updated its guidelines for prostate cancer detection. Because the current evidence about the value of testing for early prostate cancer detection is insufficient to recommend that average-risk men undergo regular screening (96), the ACS recommendations emphasize the importance of shared decision-making about testing. The ACS further recommends that the PSA blood test and DRE be offered annually beginning at age 50 years to men who have a life expectancy of at least 10 years and that a discussion take place about the potential benefits, limitations, and harms associated with testing (Table 1). In men in whom DRE is an obstacle to testing, PSA alone is an acceptable alternative.

Men at high risk, including men of sub-Saharan African descent and men with a first-degree relative diagnosed at a younger age (i.e., less than 65 years), should begin testing at age 45 years (41). Men at even higher risk of prostate cancer due to more than one first-degree relative diagnosed with prostate cancer before age 65 years could begin testing at age 40 years, although if the PSA is less than 1.0 mg/mL, no additional testing is needed until age 45 years. For PSAs greater than 1.0 mg/mL but less than 2.5 mg/mL, annual testing is recommended. If the PSA is 2.5 mg/mL or greater, further evaluation with biopsy should be considered.

There is a relatively small body of literature dealing with prostate cancer in HIV-infected men (97,98). As mentioned earlier in this chapter, among 1142 ELPWAs, prostate cancer risk was low overall (RR = 0.8), perhaps because of reduced screening in that cohort (15). Whether this is due to lack of an association or inadequate screening is unclear (99). Prostate cancer has been reported in HIV-positive men older than 60 years with chronic HIV infection and relatively preserved CD4+ cell counts (100).

To determine the incidence of prostate cancer in men with HIV infection, researchers at the Naval Medical Center in San Diego screened HIV-infected men for prostate carcinoma (100). They monitored PSA levels and included a DRE as part of routine annual health maintenance provided to HIV-positive men older than 35 years. Among 269 patients, seven (2.6%) had an elevated PSA value and none had an abnormal DRE result. Three of these patients were diagnosed with prostatitis, one with high-grade prostatic intraepithelial neoplasia, and none with cancer.

There have been too few cases published to reliably determine the biologic behavior of prostate cancer in the HIV setting (27). To systematically evaluate the approach to management of localized prostate cancer in HIV-positive patients in the HAART era, researchers at Columbia University in New York initiated a retrospective analysis of 10 HIV-positive patients with clinically localized prostate cancer (101). The average patient was 54 years old, had been HIV positive for nine years, and had a CD4+ T-lymphocyte count of 417 cells/µL, a PSA level of 9.2 mg/mL, and a Gleason score of 6. Eight patients had risk factors for prostate cancer (African-American descent, positive family history). These HIV-positive patients were treated with prostatectomy, brachytherapy, external beam radiotherapy, and/or hormonal treatment.

Until we know more about the incidence and natural history of prostate cancer in the setting of HIV infection, consider applying prostate cancer screening guidelines for HIV-infected patients in a manner and frequency that is customary for non-HIV-infected individuals.

CONCLUSIONS

Since the introduction of HAART, significant shifts have occurred in the frequency and clinical presentation of AIDS-defining conditions and AIDS-related deaths. Improvements in life expectancy of patients with HIV make it possible and important to evaluate and plan for the long-term health maintenance of these individuals.

In recent years, age at the time of diagnosis of AIDS has progressively increased. In the United States, 10% to 15% of AIDS cases are diagnosed in individuals older than 50 years, and a consistent number of AIDS cases are being diagnosed in people over 65, especially in women. According to epidemiological data, it is estimated that there are presently 60,000 HIV-positive individuals older than 60 years in the United States (102). In the general population, most common tumors (e.g., lung, breast, prostate, and colorectal cancer) increase exponentially over 50 years of age, and rates of the most common types of cancer in the elderly can be expected to also increase in the near future as HIV-positive individuals grow older. For this group, the impact of HAART on cancer incidence rates is still to be defined.

The problems connected with non-ADMs, including early-diagnosis methods and procedures for the most common of neoplasms, have not been well publicized. An important first step is to prevent the occurrence of cancer through tobacco cessation efforts (103). Furthermore, the compliance of HIV-positive individuals with early cancer diagnosis programs must be evaluated: screening is now available for a population cohort before disease symptoms occur.

For EPWAs, comprehensive medical care must include specific cancer screening and early diagnosis programs. The time has come to investigate the relation among HIV infection, age, and cancer (103). These studies may produce new findings with reference to the natural history of HIV infection and give us new opportunities to improve the overall clinical treatment of HIV-positive individuals.

REFERENCES

1. Centers for Disease Control. 1993 revised clarification system for HIV infection and expanded surveillance case definition for AIDS among adolescents and adults. MMWR Recomm Rep 1992; 41(RR17):1–19.
2. Chang Y, Cesarman E, Pessin M, et al. Identification of herpesvirus-like DNA sequences in AIDS-associated Kaposi's sarcoma. Science 1994; 266:1865–1869.
3. Epstein MA, Achong BG, Barr Y. Virus particles in cultured lymphoblasts from Burkitt's lymphoma. Lancet 1964; 1:702–703.
4. Zur Hausen H. Papillomaviruses in human cancer. Appl Pathol 1987; 5:19–24.
5. Grulich AE, van Leeuwen MT, Falster MO, et al. Incidence of cancers in people with HIV/AIDS compared with immunosuppressed transplant recipients: a meta-analysis. Lancet 2007; 370:59–67.
6. Highly active antiretroviral therapy and incidence of cancer in human immunodeficiency virus-infected adults. International Collaboration on HIV and Cancer. J Natl Cancer Inst 2000; 92:1823–1830.
7. Hessol NA, Pipkin S, Schwarcz S, et al. The impact of highly active antiretroviral therapy on non-AIDS defining cancers among adults with AIDS. Am J Epidemiol 2007; 165:1143–1553.
8. Herida A, Mary-Krause M, Kaphan R, et al. Incidence of non-AIDS-defining cancers before and during the highly active antiretroviral therapy era in a cohort of human-immunodeficiency virus-infected patients. J Clin Oncol 2003; 21:3447–3453.
9. Clifford GM, Polesel J, Rickenbach M, et al. Cancer risk in the Swiss HIV cohort: associations with immunodeficiency, smoking, and highly active antiretroviral therapy. J Natl Cancer Inst 2005; 97:425–432.
10. Detels R, Tarwater P, Phair JP, et al. For the Multicenter AIDS Cohort Study. Effectiveness of potent antiretroviral therapies on the incidence of opportunistic infections before and after AIDS diagnosis. AIDS 2001; 15:347–355.
11. Sterne JA, Hernan MA, Ledergerber B, et al. For the Swiss HIV Cohort Study. Long term effectiveness of potent antiretroviral therapy in preventing AIDS and death: a prospective cohort study. Lancet 2005; 366:378–384.
12. Smit C, Geskus R, Walker S, et al. For the Cascade Collaboration. Effective therapy has altered the spectrum of cause-specific mortality following HIV seroconversion. AIDS 2006; 20:741–749.
13. Biggar RJ, Chaturvedi AK, Goedert JJ, et al. For the HIV/AIDS Cancer Match Study. AIDS-related cancer and severity of immunosuppression in persons with AIDS. J Natl Cancer Inst 2007; 99:962–972.

14. Sackoff JE, Hanna DB, Pfeiffer MR, et al. Causes of death among persons with AIDS in the era of highly active antiretroviral therapy: New York City. Ann Intern Med 2006; 145:397–406.
15. Biggar RJ, Kirby KA, Atkinson J, et al. For the AIDS Cancer Match Study Group. Cancer risk in elderly persons with HIV/AIDS. J Acquir Immune Defic Syndr 2004; 36:861–868.
16. Palella FJ Jr., Baker RK, Moorman AC, et al. Mortality in the highly active antiretroviral therapy era: changing causes of death and disease in the HIV outpatient study. J Acquir Immune Defic Syndr 2006; 43:27–34.
17. Bonnet F, Lewden C, May T, et al. Malignancy-related causes of death in human immunodeficiency virus-infected patients in the era of highly active antiretroviral therapy. Cancer 2004; 101:317–324.
18. American Cancer Society. Cancer Facts and Figures 2005. Atlanta: American Cancer Society 2005.
19. Hessol NA, Seaberg EC, Preston-Martin S, et al. Cancer risk among participants of the Women's Interagency HIV Study. J. Acquir Immune Defic Syndr 2004; 36:978–985.
20. Armitage P, Doll R. The age distribution of cancer and a multi-stage theory of carcinogenesis. Br J Cancer 1954; 8:1–12.
21. Engels EA. Human immunodeficiency virus infection, aging, and cancer. J Clin Epidemiol 2001; 54(suppl 1):S29–S34.
22. Barbaro G, Barbarini G. HIV infection and cancer in the era of highly active antiretroviral therapy (Review). Oncol Reports 2007; 17:1121–1126.
23. Moubayed P, Mwakyoma H, Schneider DT. High frequency of human papilloma virus 6/11, 16, and 18 infections in precancerous lesions and squamous cell carcinoma of the conjunctiva in subtropical Tanzania. Am J Cln Pathol 2004; 122:938–943.
24. Ateenyi-Agaba C, Dai M, Le Calvez F, et al. TP 53 mutations in squamous-cell carcinomas of the conjunctiva: evidence of UV-induced mutagenesis. Mutagenesis 2004; 19:399–401.
25. Kew MC. Hepatitis B and C viruses and hepatocellular carcinoma. Clin Lab Med 1996; 16:395–406.
26. Sterling RK, Sulkowski MS. Hepatitis C virus in the setting of HIV or hepatitis B virus coinfection. Semin Liv Dis 2004; 24(suppl 2):61–68.
27. Pantanowitz L, Schecht HP, Dezube BJ. The growing problem of non-AIDS-defining malignancies in HIV. Curr Opin Oncol 2006; 18:469–478.
28. Gulick RM, Su Z, Flexner C, et al. Phase 2 study of the safety and efficacy of Vicriviroc, a CCR5 inhibitor, in HIV-1 infected treatment-experienced patients: AIDS Clinical Trials Group 5211. J Infect Dis 2007; 196:304–312.
29. Braithwaite RS, Justice AC, Change CC, et al. Estimating the proportion of patients infected with HIV who will die of comorbid diseases. Am J Med 2005; 118: 890–898.
30. Crothers K, Griffith TA, McGinnis KA, et al. The impact of cigarette smoking on mortality, quality of life, and comorbid illness among HIV-positive veterans. J Gen Intern Med 2005; 20:1142–1445.
31. Justice AC, Lasky E, McGinnis KA. Medical disease and alcohol use among veterans with human immunodeficiency virus infection: a comparison of disease measurement strategies. Med Care 2006; 44(8 suppl 2):S52–S60.
32. Engels EA, Pfeiffer RM, Goedert JJ, et al. Trends in cancer risk among people with AIDS in the United States 1980–2002. AIDS 2006; 20:1645–1654.

33. Spano JP, Massiani MA, Bentata M, et al. Lung cancer in patients with HIV infection and review of the literature. Med Oncol 2004; 21:109–115.
34. Kirk GD, Merlo C, O'Driscoll P, et al. HIV infection is associated with an increased risk for lung cancer, independent of smoking. Clin Infect Dis 2007; 45:103–110.
35. Chaturvedi AK, Pfeiffer RM, Chang L, et al. Elevated risk of lung cancer among people with AIDS. AIDS 2007; 21:207–213.
36. International collaboration on HIV and Cancer. Highly active antiretroviral therapy and incidence of cancer in human immunodeficiency virus-infected adults. J Natl Cancer Inst 2000; 92:1823–1830.
37. Thio CL, Seabert EC, Skolasky R Jr., et al. HIV-1, hepatitis B virus, and risk of liver-related mortality in the Multicenter Cohort Study (MACS). Lancet 2002; 360:1921–1926.
38. Darby SC, Ewart DW, Giangrande PL, et al. Mortality from liver cancer and liver disease in haemophilic men and boys in UK given blood products contaminated with hepatitis C. UK Haemophilia Center Directors' Organisation. Lancet 1997; 350:1425–1431.
39. Silverberg MJ, Newhaus J, Bauer M, et al. Risk of cancers during interrupted antiretroviral therapy in the SMART Study. AIDS 2007; 21;1957–1963.
40. May MT, Sterne JA, Costagliola D, et al. HIV treatment response and prognosis in Europe and North America in the first decade of highly active antiretroviral therapy: a collaborative analysis. Lancet 2006; 368:451–458.
41. Smith RA, Cokkindes V, Eyre HJ. Cancer screening in the United States: 2007: a review of current guidelines, practices, and prospects. CA Cancer J Clin 2007; 57:90–104.
42. Henschke CI, Yankelevitz DF, Libby DM, et al. Survival of patients with stage I lung cancer detected on CT screening. N Engl J Med 2006; 355:1763–1771.
43. American College of Obstetricians and Gynecologists. Recommendations for women's health screening and care. Available at: http://www.acog.org/.
44. New York Health Department. Primary care approach to the HIV-infected patient. 2007.
45. Parkin DM, Bray F, Ferlay J, et al. Global cancer statistics, 2002. CA Cancer J Clin 2005; 55:74–108.
46. Kosary CL. FIGO stage, histology, histologic grade, age and race as prognostic factors in determining survival for cancers of the female gynecological system: an analysis of 1973–87 SEER cases of cancers of the endometrium, cervix, ovary, vulva, and vagina. Semin Surg Oncol 1994; 10:31–46.
47. Monk BJ, Tewari KS, Koh WJ. Multimodality therapy for locally advanced cervical carcinoma: state of the art and future directions. J Cln Oncol 2007; 25:2952–2965.
48. Wright TC Jr., Schiffman M, Solomon D, et al. Interim guidance for the use of human papillomavirus DNA testing as a adjunct to cervical cytology for screening. Obstet Gynecol 2004; 103:304–309.
49. Kojic EM, Cu-Uvin S. Human papillomavirus (HPV) infection of the anus is more prevalent and diverse than cervical HPV infection among HIV-infected women in the SUN study. 44th Annual Meeting of the Infectious Disease Society of America. Toronto, October 12–15, 2006; Abstract 693.
50. Highleyman L, Human Papillomavirus. BETA, Summer 2007:35–39.
51. Plummer M, Schiffman M, Castle PE, et al. For the ALTS group. A 2-year prospective study of human papillomavirus persistence among women with a

cytological diagnosis of atypical squamous cells of undetermined significance or low-grade squamous intraepithelial lesion. J Infect Dis 2007; 195:1582–1589.

52. Palefsky JM. Human papillomavirus infection in HIV-infected persons. Top HIV Med 2007; 15:130–133.
53. Maiman M, Fruchter RG, Sedlis A, et al. Prevalence, risk factors, and accuracy of cytological screening for cervical intraepithelial neoplasia in women with human immunodeficiency virus infection. Gynecol Oncol 1998; 68:233–239.
54. Womack SD, Chirenje ZM, Gaffiken L, et al. HPV-based cervical cancer screening in a population at high risk for HIV infection. Int J Cancer 2000; 85:206–210.
55. Delmas MC, Larsen C, Van Benthem B, et al. Cervical squamous intraepithelial lesions in HIV-infected women: prevalence, incidence, and regression. European Study Group on national history of HIV infection in women. AIDS 2000; 14:1775–1784.
56. Heard I, Tassie JM, Schmitz V, et al. Increased risk of cervical disease among human immunodeficiency virus-infected women with severe immunosuppression and high human papillomavirus load. Obstet Gynecol 2000; 96:403–409.
57. Harris TG, Burd RD, Palefsky JM, et al. Incidence of cervical squamous intra-epithelial lesions associated with HIV serostatus, CD4 cell counts, and human papillomavirus test results. JAMA 2005; 293:1471–1476.
58. Chirenje ZM. HIV and Cancer of the Cervix. Best Prac Res Clin Obstet Gynaecol 2005; 19:269–276.
59. Heard I, Tassie JM, Kazatchkine MD, et al. Highly active antiretroviral therapy enhances regression of cervical intraepithelial neoplasia in HIV-seropositive women. AIDS 2002; 16:1799–1802.
60. Moore AL, Sabin CA, Madge S, et al. Highly active antiretroviral therapy and cervical intraepithelial neoplasia. AIDS 2002; 16:927–929.
61. Piketty C, Kazatchkine MD. Human papillomavirus-related cervical and anal disease in HIV-infected individuals in the era of highly active antiretroviral therapy. Curr HIV/AIDS Rep 2005; 2:140–145.
62. Kojic EM, Cu-Uvin S. Special care issues of women living with HIV-AIDS. Infect Dis Clin N Am 2007; 21:133–148.
63. Franceshi S, Jaffe H. Cervical cancer screenings of women living with HIV infection: a must in the era of antiretroviral therapy. Clin Infect Dis 2007; 45:510–513.
64. Johnson ZG, Madeleine MM, Newcomer LM, et al. Anal cancer incidence and survival, epidemiology, and end results experience, 1973–2000. Cancer 2004; 101:281–288.
65. Daling JR, Weiss NS, Hislop TG, et al. Sexual practices, sexually transmitted diseases, and the incidence of anal cancer. N Engl J Med 1987; 317:973–977.
66. Goedert JJ, Coté TR, Virgo P, et al. Spectrum of AIDS-associated malignant disorders. Lancet 1998; 351:1833–1839.
67. Bower M, Powles T, Newscom-Davis T, et al. HIV-associated anal cancer: has highly active antiretroviral therapy reduced the incidence or improved the outcome? J Acquir Immune Defic Syndr 2004; 37:1563–1565.
68. Diamond C, Taylor TH, Aboumrad T, et al. Increased incidence of squamous cell anal cancer among men with AIDS in the era of highly active antiretroviral therapy. Sex Trasm Dis 2005; 32:314–320.
69. Bjorge T, Engerland A, Luostarinen T, et al. Human papillomavirus infection as a risk factor for anal and perianal skin cancer in a prospective study. Br J Cancer 2002; 87:61–64.

70. Chiao EY, Giordano TP, Palefsky JM, et al. Screening HIV-infected individuals for anal cancer precursor lesions: a systematic review. Cln Infect Dis 2006; 43:223–233.
71. Kim JH, Sarani B, Orkin BA, et al. HIV-positive patients with anal carcinoma have poorer treatment tolerance and outcome than HIV-negative patients. Dis Colon Rectum 2001; 44:1496–1502.
72. Chin-Hong PV, Vittinghoff E, Cranston RD, et al. Age-related prevalence of anal cancer precursors in homosexual men: The EXPLORE Study. J Natl Cancer Inst 2005; 97:896–905.
73. Abramowitz L, Benabderrahmane D, Ravaud P, et al. Anal squamous intraepithelial lesions and condyloma in HIV-infected heterosexual men, homosexual men and women: prevalence and associated factors. AIDS 2007; 21:1457–1465.
74. Fox PA, Seet JA, Stebbing J, et al. The value of anal cytology and human papillomavirus typing in the detection of anal intraepithelial neoplasia: a review of cases from an anoscopy clinic. Sex Transm Infect 2005; 81:142–146.
75. Cranston RD, Hart SD, Gornbein JA, et al. The prevalence, and predictive value, of abnormal anal cytology to diagnose anal dysplasia in a population of HIV-positive men who have sex with men. Int J of STD AIDS 2007; 18:77–80.
76. Lampinen TM, Latulippe L, van Niekerk D, et al. Illustrated instructions for self-collection of anorectal swab specimens and their adequacy for cytological examination. Sex Transm Dis 2006; 33:386–388.
77. Berry JM, Palefsky JM, Welton ML. Anal cancer and its precursors in HIV-positive patients: perspectives and management. Surg Oncol Clin N Am 2004; 13:355–373.
78. Chin-Hong PV, Palefsky JM. Natural history and clinical management of anal human papillomavirus disease in men and women infected with human immunodeficiency virus. Clin Infect Dis 2002; 35:1127–1134.
79. Jemal A, Murray T, Ward E, et al. Cancer Statistics, 2005. CA Cancer J Clin 2005; 55:10–30.
80. Pignone M, Rich M, Tuetsch SM, et al. Screening for colorectal cancer in adults at average risk: a summary of the evidence for the U.S. Preventive Services Task Force. Ann Intern Med 2002; 137:132–141.
81. Winawer S, Fletcher R, Rex D, et al. Colorectal cancer screening and surveillance: clinical guidelines and rationale – Update based on new evidence. Gastroenterology 2003; 124:544–560.
82. Bedimo R, Chen RY, Accortt NA, et al. Trends in AIDS-defining and non-AIDS-defining malignancies among HIV-infected patients: 1989–2002. Cln Infect Dis 2004; 39:1380–1384.
83. Wasserberg N, Nunoo-Mensah JW, Gonzalez-Ruiz C, et al. Colorectal cancer in HIV-infected patients: a case control study. Int J Colorectal Dis 2007; 22:1217–1221.
84. Demopoulos BP, Vamvakas E, Ehrlich JE, et al. Non-acquired immune deficiency syndrome-defining malignancies in patients infected with human immunodeficiency virus. Arch Pathol Lab Med 2003; 127:589–592.
85. Yeguez JF, Martinez SA, Sands DR, et al. Colorectal malignancies in HIV-positive patients. Am Surg 2003; 69:981–987.
86. Reinhold JP, Moon M, Tenner CT, et al. Colorectal cancer screening in HIV-infected patients 50 years of age and older: missed opportunities for prevention. Am J Gastroenterol 2005; 100:1805–1812.

87. Bini EJ, Park J, Francois F. Use of flexible sigmoidoscopy to screen for colorectal cancer in HIV-infected patients 50 years of age and older. Arch Intern Med 2006; 166:1626–1631.

88. Jemal A, Siegel R, Ward E, et al. Cancer Statistics 2007. CA Cancer J Clin 2007; 57:43–66.

89. Saslow D, Boetes C, Burke W, et al. American Cancer Society guidelines for breast screening with MRI as an adjunct to mammography. CA Cancer J Clin 2007; 57:75–89.

90. Oluwole SF, Ali AO, Shafaee Z, et al. Breast cancer in women with HIV/AIDS: report of five cases with a review of the literature. J Surg Oncol 2005; 89:23–27.

91. Gewurz BE, Dezube BJ, Pantanowitz L. HIV and the breast. AIDS Read 2005; 15:399–402.

92. Gail MH, Constantino JP, Bryant J, et al. Weighing the risks and benefits of tamoxifen treatment for preventing breast cancer. J Natl Cancer Inst 1999; 91: 1829–1846.

93. Seth AN, Moore RD, Gebo KA. Provision of general and HIV-specific health maintenance in middle aged adults and older patients in an urban HIV clinic. AIDS Patient Care STDs 2006; 20:318–325.

94. Preston-Martin S, Kirstein LM, Pogoda JM, et al. Use of mammographic screening by HIV-infected women in the Women's Interagency HIV Study (WIHS). Prev Med 2002; 34:386–392.

95. Walter LC, Bertenthal D, Lindquist K, et al. PSA screening among elderly men with limited life expectancies. JAMA, 2006; 296:2336–2342.

96. Nam RK, Toi A, Klotz LH, et al. Assessing individual risk for prostate cancer. J Cln Oncol 2007; 25:3582–3588.

97. Furco A, Bani-Sader F, Guymar S, et al. Metastatic cancer of the prostate in a young 40 year-old HIV-infected male patient. Presse Med 2003; 32:930–931.

98. Quatan N, Nair S, Harrowes F, et al. Should HIV patients be considered a high risk group for the development of prostate cancer? Am R Coll Surg Engl 2005; 87: 437–438.

99. Crum NF, Hale B, Utz G, et al. Increased risk of prostate cancer in HIV infection? AIDS 2002; 16:1703–1704.

100. Crum NF, Spencer CR, Amling CL. Prostate carcinoma among men with human immunodeficiency virus infection. Cancer 2004; 101:294–299.

101. Levinson A, Nagler EA, Lowe FC. Approach to management of clinically localized prostate cancer in patients with human immunodeficiency virus. Urology 2005; 65:91–94.

102. Linsk NL. HIV among older adults: age specific issues in prevention and treatment. AIDS Read 2000; 10:430–440.

103. di Gennaro G, Cinelli R, Vaccher E, et al. Cancer prevention and early diagnosis in HIV-positive individuals. J Acquir Immune Defic Syndr 2005; 38:628–629.

Index

DATE DUE